THE 23 PILLARS OF ESOTERIC GERONTOLOGY

How To End Aging

Other Books by Duke Watrous

HOW TO RAISE A
RUGGED INDIVIDUALIST
-a father's perspective

WHAT'S IN A LIFE
The Duke Watrous Story

Mind Mechanics
How to Create your
Conscious Experience
Find Success, Find Purpose, & Find Happiness

Space Colony
A Novel About the Future

Moving?
A Guide to Hiring a Moving Company
and/or Moving yourself

THE 23 PILLARS OF ESOTERIC GERONTOLOGY

How To End Aging

By

Duke Watrous

Books may be purchased in quantity and/or special sales by contacting the publisher by email at duke@dukewatrous.com

Published by: Create Space
Photos By: DepositPhotos.com, and Author
Interior Design by: Duke Watrous
Cover Design by: Duke Watrous
Copy Editing by: Kasidee Rumsey
Watrous, Duke 1973-

The 23 Pillars Of
Esoteric Gerontology

Library of Congress
**ISBN-13:
978-1978058835**

**ISBN-10:
1978058837**

1. Anti-aging 2. Aging 3. **Gerontology** 4. Longevity

DEDICATION

This book is dedicated to ending aging, to every person working on extending life, to everyone who is working on a cure for aging, to anyone who does not want to die, to the philosopher who uses logic and reason to convince people that they don't have to die, and to all who have their bodies cryogenically frozen so that in the future they can be revived.

Aging is the most deadly disease that there is. It destroys the mind and makes the body decrepit. It eats away at our most precious memories, and it destroys our families.

It kills our loved ones, and no one even blames it. It steals our beauty and strength, and it destroys our ambitions, hopes, and dreams.

After aging has done all this, we give it a pass, and act like growing old is desirable or romantic.

We will overcome the greatest scourge on humankind. We will destroy the greatest genocide the world has ever known; we will find a cure for aging!

Duke Watrous

THE 23 PILLARS OF ESOTERIC GERONTOLOGY

1. Sleep And Recovery
2. Hydration, Detoxification, Inflammation, And Oxidation
3. Diet And Nutrition
4. Nutraceuticals
5. Hormone Balance
6. Exercise
7. Regenerative Medicine
8. Hypothermic Protocol
9. Artificial Implants And Nano Technology
10. Genomics, Gene Therapy, And Gene Expression
11. Stem Cell Colonies And Stem Cell Reseeding
12. Immunosenescence
13. General Senescence
14. Cell Loss And Cell Atrophy
15. Telomeres
16. Mitochondria Mutations
17. Advanced Glycation End Products And Protein Cross Links
18. Intercellular Junk, Lipofuscin Build Up
19. Extra Cellular Junk And Misshapen Proteins
20. DNA Mutations And Cancer
21. Old Age Brain Diseases
22. New Diseases And Proactive Research
23. Cryonics Arrangements

ACKNOWLEDGMENTS

Smart men and women
that write brilliant books.
People that are visionaries, people
that see the world not as is could be,
but as it should be.

.

THE 23 PILLARS OF ESOTERIC GERONTOLOGY

Gerontology is the scientific study of aging. Esoteric is intended or understood by a small group with specialized knowledge or interests. Esoteric Gerontology is the study of aging by a small interested group of people with specialized knowledge who have the intention of dramatically extending the human life span.

The founding premise of Esoteric Gerontology is that aging is a disease, and as a disease it can be cured. Diseases must be studied, analyzed, models created, hypotheses tested, and cures implemented.

Aging is a disease that affects nearly all body functions. No one that we know of has escaped the debilitating effects of this disease. Every one that has lived long enough dies of old age, or so we believe. People that die of old age actually die of a malfunction of an organ or bodily system, but it is said to be old age. The ravages of aging are well understood and affect humans at a predictable rate. Doctors tell us that we are "healthy for our age."

Getting old has been romanticized and even embraced. Young lovers telling each other, "I want to grow old with you." Wrinkles and gray hair are a mark of distinguishment, a good life with the natural conclusion being death. I even read: "Appealing as the idea of lengthening the human lifespan may be, some find it deeply disturbing. We already live long enough, they argue. There are too many people on the planet now, and living beyond a normal lifespan would be selfish. Besides, death is a natural part of life, and gives it its meaning," *(Redesigning Humans: Choosing Our Genes, Changing Our Future, 79).*

I once heard life described as a collection of moments, each moment as precious as a diamond. If we had fields of diamonds, they would lose their value. What makes life so precious is we only have so much time. In other words, life is valuable because of the scarcity principle.

Most philosophers today and religious leaders value death as a means of measuring life. When popular fiction addresses extreme long life or immortality, it is seen a burden, a curse. The man that has lived hundreds of years yearns for the sweet release of death.

The inevitable march toward death seems to most people to be self-evident, so people accept death. But not really. Death is psychologically impossible to reconcile in the human mind. People deny death. People avoid death. People ignore death. People build complex cognitive constructs to deal with their own and their loved one's mortality.

Romanticizing and waxing poetic about our

mortality does nothing to protect us from the cold hard facts that aging is killing us. An enemy recognized, is an enemy half defeated. Today few people will acknowledge that death is our greatest enemy.

This has not always been so. Humanity has a rich history of acknowledging that death is our enemy. The Epic of Gilgamesh tells of an ancient king and his quest for immortality. The Holy Grail and the fountain of youth, drink and the clock of aging is reversed. It seems that almost every culture has a myth or legend of some adventurer seeking to shortchange death. We also learn that immortality without youth means little. What good is living a long time if you are too sick to enjoy it? Long life needs to be accompanied by good health.

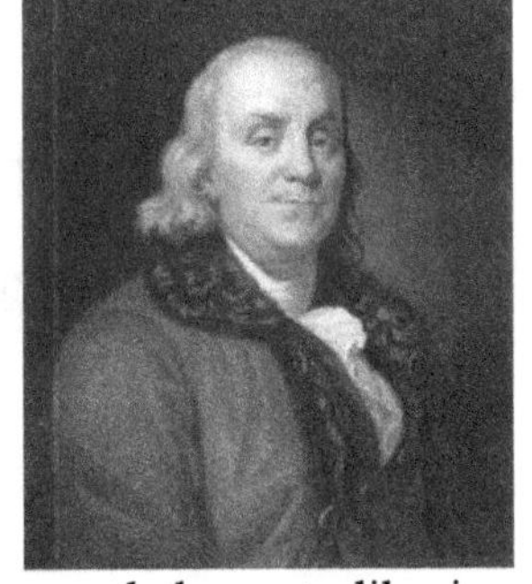

"All diseases may by sure means be prevented or cured not excepting even that of old age and our life lengthened at pleasure, even beyond the antediluvian standard." -Benjamin Franklin

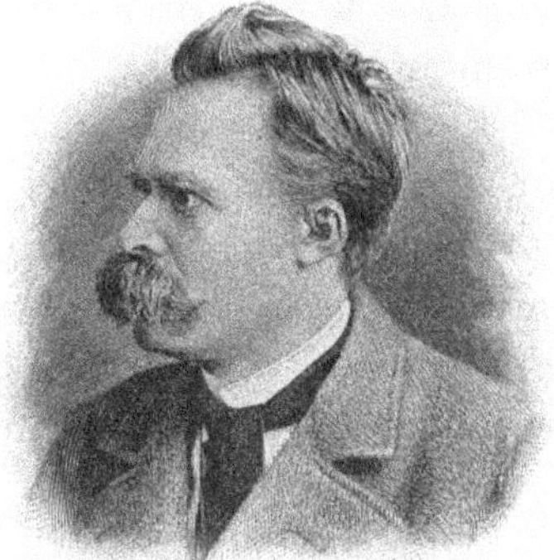

Friedrich Nietzsche.

"Is life not a thousand times too short for us to bore ourselves?" -Nietzsche

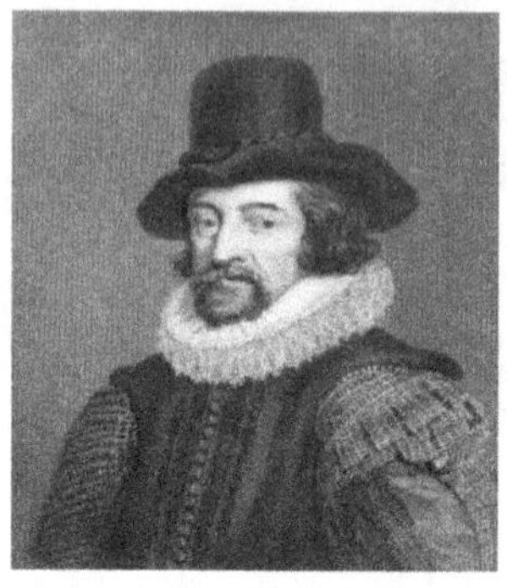

"Whatever can be repaired gradually without destroying the original whole is, like the vestal fire, potentially eternal."   -Francis Bacon

"Death is psychologically unbearable. People deal with it in different ways. The four main categories are:

1. Denial - "Just don't think about it." "The future does not affect me now." "Contemplating mortality only depresses me, so let's talk about something else."

2. Belief in an After Life - Churches fill pews with their threats and promises of what their God will do with you when you die.

3. Unrealistic Thinking - "I will be so healthy, I just won't die." This is a variation of "denial." Some transhumanists, cryonics members, immoralists, and radical life extensionists, are trying to achieve actual immortality like King Gilgamesh of ancient Sumer. Chasing after the "fountain of youth".

4. Leave a Legacy - Leave your mark on this world. Build things, invent things, create art, write books, et cetera. People put their names on things to be remembered (e.g., bridges, ships, cities, buildings, libraries, businesses, foundations, streets and freeways, farm and ranch entrances). Your kiddos are your genetic legacy," (*How to Raise a Rugged Individualist - a father's perspective*, chapter 36).

People can be a slave to their culture and their beliefs. Almost every advance and discovery has been laughed at and ridiculed. "The Earth is the center of the universe." "The earth is flat." "If God wanted man to fly, he would have given him wings." "There will never be space travel." "Anesthesia, antibiotics, vaccinations, et cetera, we don't need them. That's playing God."

The new technologies and discoveries go through three stages:

1. Mocked and laughed at. "It will never work."
2. Opposed, sometimes with violence.
3. Accepted as self-evident.

I don't care that society at large thinks extending the human lifespan to 150 and beyond is ridiculous. Provided people leave people alone to pursue their own goals, it will matter little. My concern is that people like to force their agenda on other people. Whether forcing conversion to a religion at the point of a sword/gun, or legally preventing people from taking anti-aging medications and cures, both are a violation of our fundamental human rights. Under natural law we can do what we want with our own lives and our own bodies. When governments issue decrees in the name of what is best for us, they are really saying that the government owns us and that we are not freemen, but property.

Is there a precedent for extended life? Nature does have some long lived life forms. There is a bristle cone pine that is over 5062 years old, lobsters have lived over 100 years, Rougheye

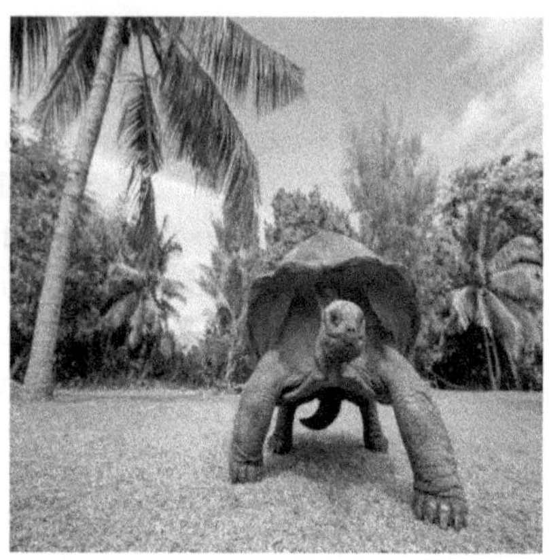

rockfish can live over 205, there is a giant tortoise, named Adwaita, that died at 255 years, ocean quahog clams have been observed as old as 507 years, and they found a two-meter Greenland shark that would be older than George Washington, if he were alive today.

The Jellyfish Turritopsis dohrnii is biologically immortal. The adult can convert back to its baby form through a process known as trans-differentiation.

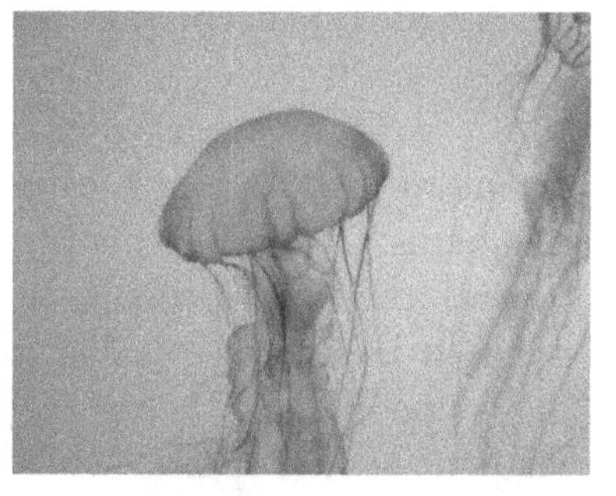

In the lab, selective breeding of fruit flies has increased their lifespan by four times. One mutation in the nematode Caenorhabditis elegans doubled its life span. If lab mice were people, their life span would have rocketed from 80 to 133 years old.

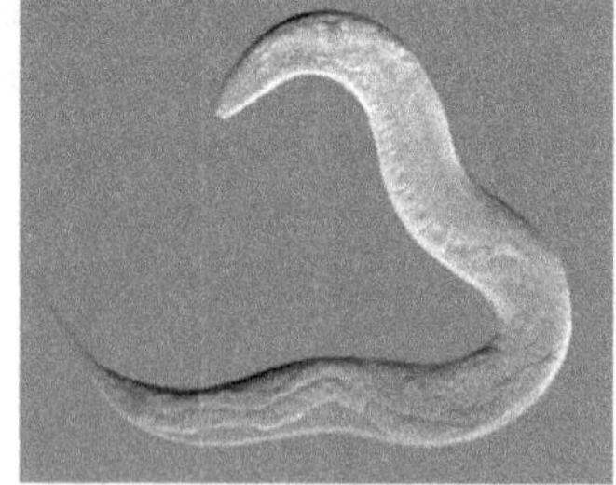

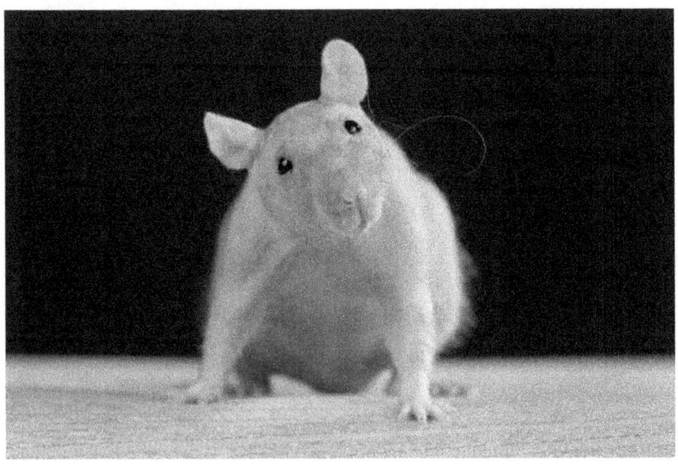

People are not animals, but all life on earth from trees to fruit flies share the same code of life, Deoxyribonucleic acid (DNA).

Never before in human history has our medical sciences been so advanced and with so much promise. Never before could we articulate the mechanisms of aging. Never before could we have a realistic conversation and design engineering methods to reverse aging.

In 2011, I read an article about Sierra sciences, and their effort to lengthen the telomeres at the end of our chromosomes. I had never heard of a telomere before, but it seemed that this was the way to put the cap on aging.

Telomeres are the section at the end of a DNA strand that holds it together. Like the plastic aglet at the end of a shoelace to keep it from unraveling. Each time the cell divides, it goes through mitosis, and the telomeres get shorter and shorter. After the Hayflick Limit is reached, the cell can't divide anymore and dies, apoptosis, or it hangs around useless, senescence. A biological marker for age is the length of your telomeres.

I read about senescent cells. Cells that for one reason or another are no longer useful, but won't go into Apoptosis, or cell suicide. Senescent cells are like zombies, toxic to other cells, useless to the body. Lots of things can turn a cell senescent: short telomeres, age, mutation, toxins, et cetera, but the main problem is that the immune system is giving them a free pass. If the zombie cell would just die or be killed, a young, fresh cell could take its place. Our immune system regularly seeks out and destroys senescent cells when things are functioning normally.

In 2011, I also read a lot about stem cells. I soon realized that a lot of the media and government propaganda misrepresented what stem cells are and what they could do.

I thought to myself, the trifecta of immortality would be, science understanding maturing telomeres, stem cells. and pulling out the senescent cells. I was soon to find out it was a bit more complicated than that.

In 2012, I read *Ending Aging* by Aubrey de Grey. Where he outlined strategies for engineered negligible senescence (SENS). Dr. de Grey argued that we did not have to cure aging. Just fix age related problems from an engineering stand point. Dr. de Grey listed seven

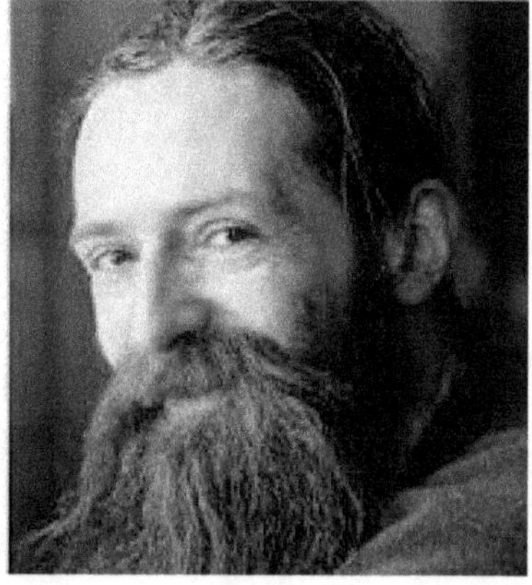

areas that needed to be addressed and fixed to stop aging so humanity could achieve what he called, "longevity escape velocity."

The SENS seven:

1. Extracellular junk, misshapen proteins that gather outside the cell that serve no purpose
2. Intracellular aggregates, lipofuscin in the lysosomes
3. Advanced glycation end products (AGEs) and protein crosslinks
4. Senescent cells
5. Mitochondrial mutations
6. Nuclear mutations
7. Cell loss and cell atrophy

Reading Dr. de Grey's book was eye opening, but more importantly, I knew that there were others. Even a community of likeminded people that love life, want to live, and understand death for what it is, a killer. People that recognize death is the end result of the disease of aging. Everyone on earth has this disease, and most consider it normal, even desirable. But there are a few people that recognize aging for what it is, and are devoting their life to finding a cure.

The biological pathways of aging at the cellular level are now better understood. For the first time in human history, technology has progressed to the point, for us as the dominant species on earth to do battle with humanity's biggest nemesis.

The medical community understands many things about what ails the human body very well. If you break a leg, any country doctor can put a cast on. If you get an infection, they can write you a prescription for antibiotics. For the most part, the 23 pillars are not about medical treatments that are widely available or broadly understood by the general public. The 23 pillars of Esoteric Gerontology are not about the short term but the dramatically extended life.

The 23 pillars are about rebuilding, replacing, and maintaining tissue and organs, and about buying the time that will make the difference. All the cells in the human body are replaced regularly, with the exception of brain and heart cells. The replacement cycle ranges from five days to seven years. If your body is operating correctly, blood, bone and flesh are all rejuvenated regularly.

Most people die from a failure of these systems of replacement and rejuvenation.

The broad theory of aging is that over time we accumulate cellular mutations and errors, that at some point reach a noticeable threshold. We begin to notice the signs of aging. One bad cell is not noticeable, but few million is.

The first six pillars are simple and can be done now. You can add thirty healthy years to your life with just the first six pillars. You can take control of your own fitness, and disease prevention. You have the power. You do not have to be a servant of medical dogma, and a prisoner of someone else's belief system.

The remaining seventeen pillars will require research, medical breakthroughs, clinical trials, and brilliant minds producing original thought. In some cases, all that is required is for the government to get out of the way. If there was a 500-page book written on government blocking medical advancements, it would just scratch the surface of all medical breakthroughs that the government has delayed or blocked. To document all of it would require a multivolume set and a team of typists.

The path to dramatically extend the human life span is before us. The areas of research are understood. The technology has been and is being developed. All that is needed is the will. An enemy recognized is an enemy half defeated. The first step is to recognize that aging is a disease. The second step is to understand the pathologies of this disease. The third step is to use the scientific method to engineer cures and treatments for the disease of aging.

There are three kinds of age.

One, your calendar age. You can find this number by looking at your driver's license, or your birth certificate. People become obsessed with their calendar age, when in reality, it is just one mark of a biological age metric.

Two, your biological age. How old you really are. How much our body has aged, is measured by our biological age, not our calendar age. I have seen forty-year-olds that look like they are sixty, a hard life, drug abuse and other factors for accelerated aging. I've seen sixty-year-olds that look like they're forty. Men and women taking care of themselves, living a healthy life, and having good genetics. We know some people die of old age in their sixties, while other people die of old age at one hundred and twenty.

Sixty years is a pretty big range to die from old age. This is why we measure our biological age, the true account of how old we really are.

Many factors go into a biological age metric. Your senescent cell load, your mitochondria health, AGEs and protein cross links, your telomere length, your bone density, your vasculature health, brain shrinkage, cell loss and cell atrophy, extracellular junk, intracellular junk, and so on. We want our biological age to be rewound to when we were in top form, perhaps late twenties or early thirties. Until radical life extension is available through future Medical Technology, we must do we can now. We can keep our biological age twenty years lower than our calendar age if we live right and take care of our mind and body. Basically, the first six pillars are about what we can do now.

Three, the maturity level. I've seen some fifty-year-olds as immature as teenagers, and I've seen some twenty-year-olds that are more mature then some senior citizens. People are different, and grow cognitively at different rates. Imagine what a maturity level could be with a couple hundred years under our belt. It is said you can judge a man by the range of his goals, the timetable of his thinking.

How much more valuable would life be if we lived one hundred, three hundred or even a thousand years? How much wisdom and experience would we command? It seems that by the time you really know how to live, you have become too old to really enjoy it. They say youth is wasted on the young. Well, let's see what an old person can do with it.

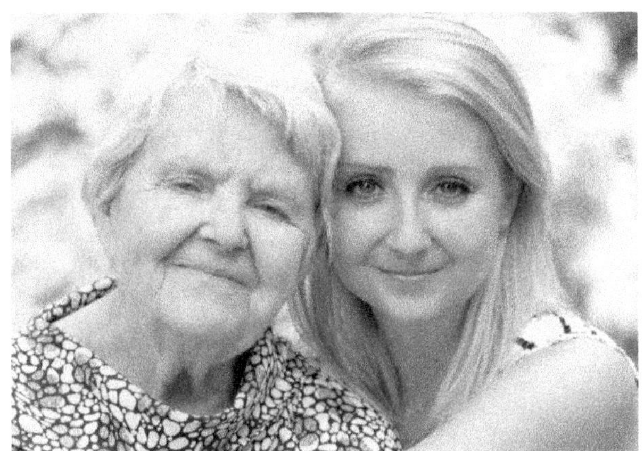

15

THE 23 PILLARS OF ESOTERIC GERONTOLOGY

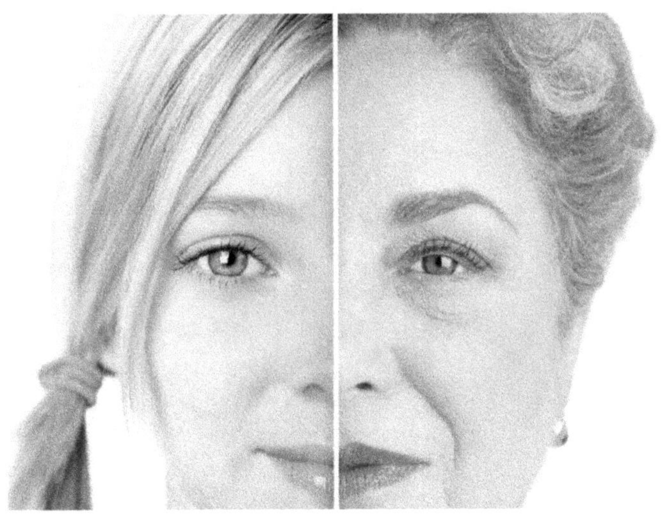

Pillar One
Sleep and Recovery.

The body's circadian rhythm affects many systems of the body. It has been shown that there are many cellular clocks that affect all kinds of operations. The main one is the sleep cycle. Poor sleep can have a cascade of negative effects: hormone cycles, repair cycles, brain maintenance and memory storage, the list goes on and on. Sleep apnea, poor sleep environment (noise, lighting, temperature, bed, et cetera), sleep disorders, and a disconnect with the solar cycle all take their toll. The proper quantity and quality for your unique needs must be found and met.

Recovery is not only about sleep. People that over tax themselves are doing long term harm. If you do not give your body the time and the nutrients it needs to recover you are causing damage. More withdrawals

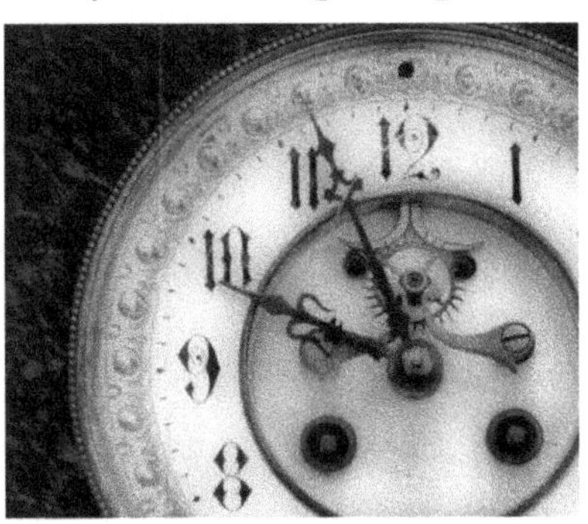

on the great balance sheet. Youth often protects us from this reality, but the debt must always be paid.

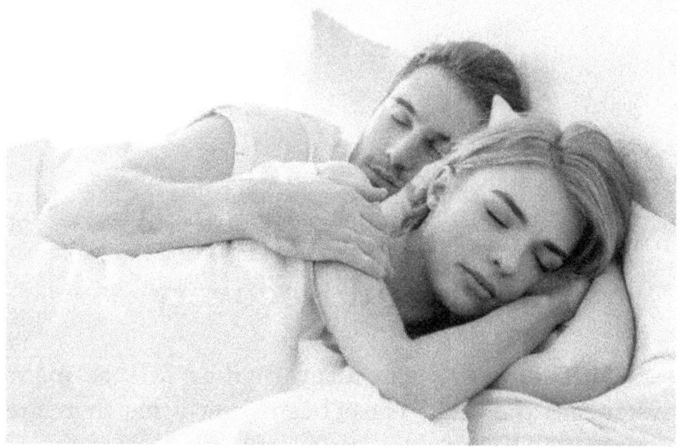

Pillar Two
Hydration, Detoxification, Inflammation, and Oxidation

Water is the universal biological solvent. The chief component of extracellular and intracellular fluid is water. All biological processes are performed in this median. Yet most people are dehydrated. The body needs clean water with the right PH in the right quantity. A lot of the water we drink is contaminated. Sometimes on purpose with fluoride and chlorine. Know what kind of water that you are drinking and drink the right amount. If you are thirsty or your urine is not clear, you are dehydrated. (yellow urine

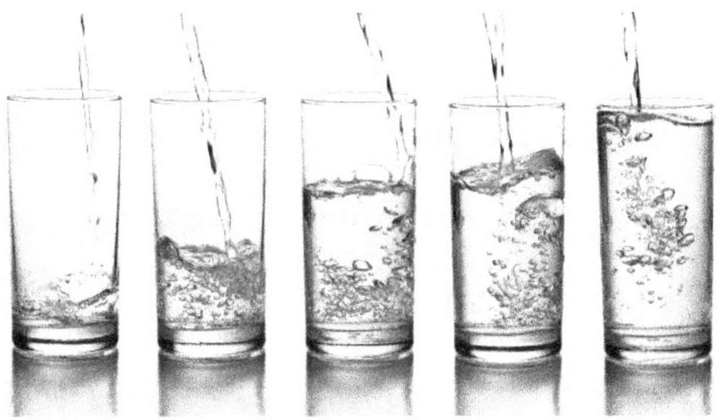

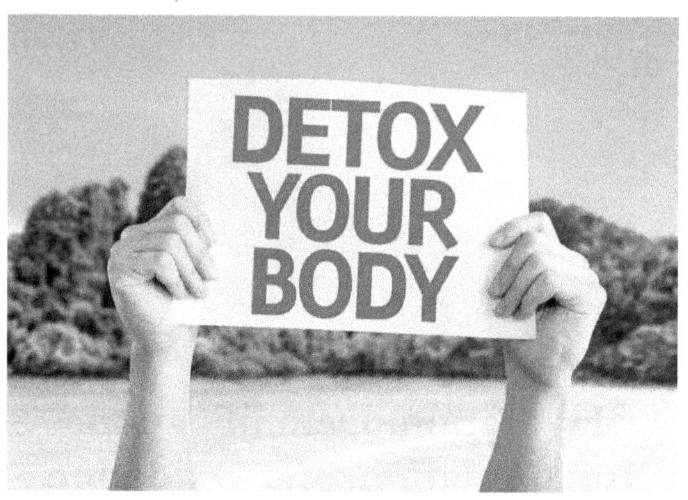

could also be caused by supplements, in that case not an indicator.)

Toxins that are absorbed through the skin, inhaled, injected, or ingested must be removed. We cannot avoid all toxins, but we can reduce our intake dramatically with life style choices.

All toxins, whether they are pesticides, exhaust fumes, drugs/alcohol, or food coloring, we must detoxify. Our kidneys and our liver do a remarkable job. Most toxins are sent out with bile, sweat, and urine. If the toxins reach levels beyond our ability to remove them, we then have build up and store the toxins in our tissue. This is a very bad thing. Not conducive to a long life. Not a big deal in the mind of a college student binge drinking, without considering their future. Know this, when toxic intake exceeds the body's ability to metabolize and pass the toxins, bad things will happen.

Inflammation is a hallmark of accelerated aging. Inflammation equals aging is about as simple as it gets. Nature intended inflammation for injury and disease on a temporary basis. Chronic inflammation causes accelerated aging. Find the causes of inflammation and stop it. Blood tests are often needed for this.

Oxidation causes accelerated aging. Limit your oxidative stress. Diet and nutraceuticals can help. Oxidation and free radicals will cause all kinds of cascades of problems in your biological processes.

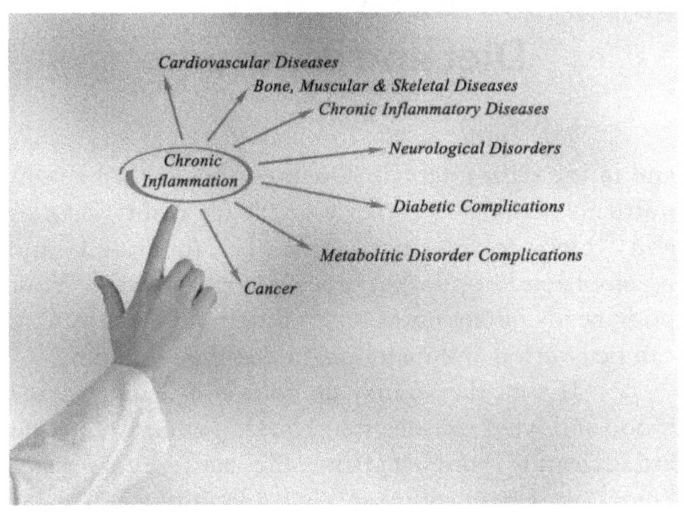

Pillar Three
Diet and Nutrition

The body needs food in the right quantities and in the right intervals. Quality foods with the right nutrients. Lots of people over fill on empty calories and toxic foods that must be processed and metabolized. Food that goes straight to fat. Your body needs ninety nutrients to function properly. You can be overfed and malnourished at the same time.

If your diet cranks up your body's detoxifying mode and what calories that you do get go to fat, you are defeating yourself from the start. People ask, "How can I be healthy, and live a long time?" I say if you are going to drive your car off a cliff, why care about what kind of motor oil to use. We are going to get into how to dramatically

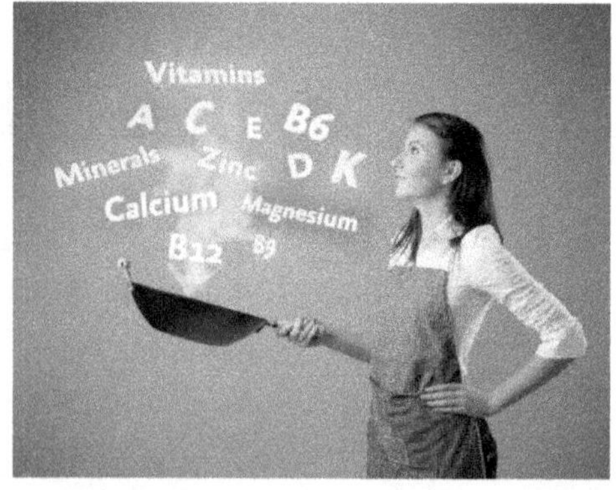

increase your life span, but if you do not care about the basics, then why even bother? Eat, drink and be merry, for tomorrow you will die. If you care about your life, then care about the basics that you can do now.

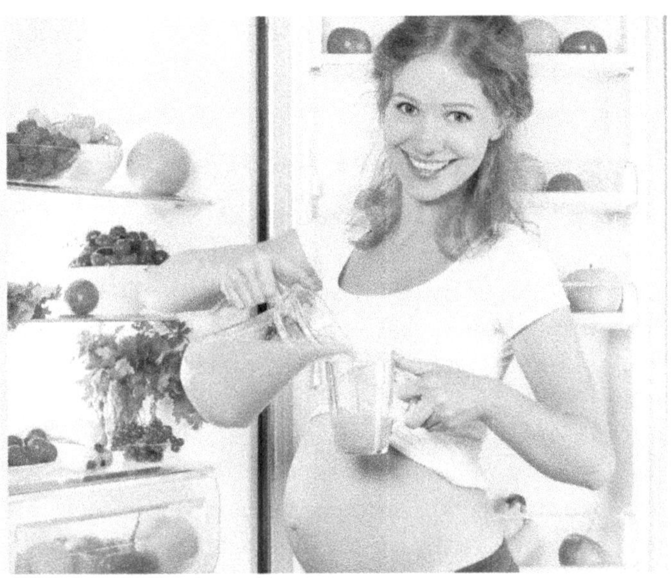

I am not saying that you have to be a health food nut. Life is about balance. Knowledge is power when is come to diet and nutrition. I would also note that eating together with the ones that you love is not only a happy part of life, but cognitively healthy as well. Break bread with the ones you love. Sharing a meal with the ones you love is happiness. Is not life about being happy?

Pillar Four
Nutraceuticals

If you can get the ninety nutrients that you need through diet, that is great, but in the real world that seldom happens. Vitamins, minerals, fatty acids, amino acids, et cetera, can all be obtained through diet but often need to be supplemented.

Each individual is unique. People absorb and retain nutrients at different rates. Blood tests are sometimes needed to assess your needs. There are a wide range of supplements with various purposes, but the basics are a benchmark for almost everyone. I recommend going to www.lifeextension.com for research and guidance.

Nutraceuticals is a study in itself. Many books have been written on this one subject, but folks still ignore the very basics of human body maintenance.

A few examples: calcium should be taken with vitamins K2, D and magnesium. Vitamin K2 is needed to bring the calcium into the collagen matrix of the bones. Vitamin D is needed to absorb calcium through the intestines. Magnesium is calcium's antagonist; calcium contracts muscles, while

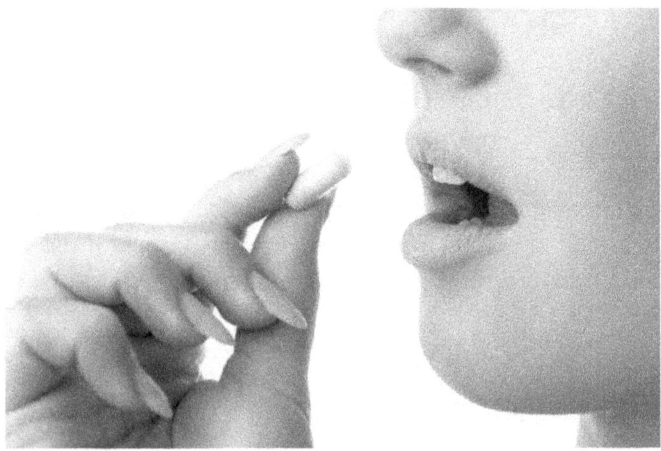

magnesium relaxes muscles.

Magnesium should be the first step in treating high blood pressure, the entire vasculature is made of smooth muscles, that relax and contract. The intracellular and extracellular fluid gradient is maintained by calcium, magnesium, potassium, and sodium. All are needed in brain function, as well. The right balance must be maintained, even the proper ratios.

We seldom hear doctors talk about electrolyte balance ratios. No, they prescribe high blood pressure medication, normally a calcium channel blocker and a diuretic (to reduce extracellular fluid volume). Vitamin K2 also helps remove calcium from the soft tissues. This reduces calcification of the arteries, wrinkles on the face, cleans the pineal gland in the brain, et cetera. If vitamin K2 can build up your bones and at the same time clean out your heart, why does the medical establishment ignore it? If magnesium deficiency is the main cause of hypertension, why is it ignored? You must do your own research; you must look out for your own body. Treat the cause of the problem, not the symptom.

Some nutrients work in synergy, like Vitamins A, D and E. Some have different forms, that can be more readily absorbed by some people. For example: chelated and attached to amino acids. Your stomach acid will destroy some nutrients, and they must be absorbed under the tongue, through the skin, or injected.

The more you know, the better decisions you can make for yourself and the ones you love.

Learning to read your own blood tests is a good idea. Give your body what it needs to be healthy. This is basic, but very important and often misunderstood. Put very simply: avoid nutrient deficiency.

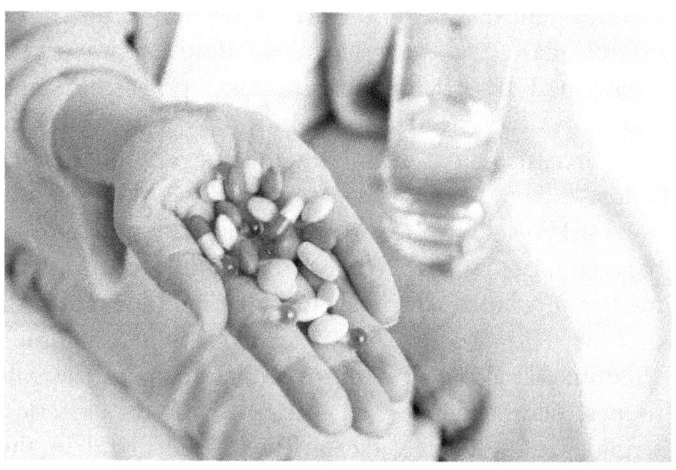

Pillar Four
Hormone Balance

Maintaining hormone balance is key to a youthful life. As we age, our hormone levels change. You can take bioidentical hormones and keep yourself at youthful levels. People literally say that they feel twenty years younger when they balance their hormones. If your doctor says that, "you are healthy for your age," that is the lepers bell to flee, and find yourself an antiaging doctor. Whatever hormone level is you at top form, is what you need to supplement to. There are people with a calendar age of seventy-five and a biological age of thirty-five, hormones are essential to this- bioidentical hormones.

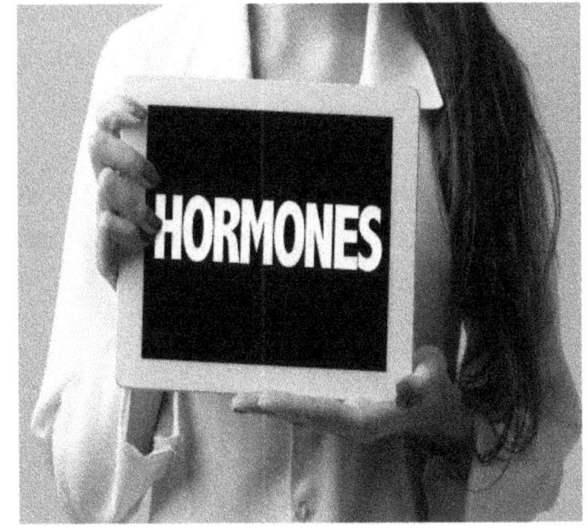

Pillar Six
Exercise

Everybody knows to exercise, this is not esoteric knowledge, but somehow people find excuses not to. Why? People are lazy, too busy, and do not understand the importance. There are as many reasons not to exercise as there are people. The reasons and excuses do not matter. Exercise is such an important key to a long life that it must be included as a pillar. The brain and the heart both have long lived cells; cells that were pumping blood and thinking when you were a baby and are still pumping blood and thinking today. The biological age of your brain and your heart is of the utmost importance.

There are four kinds of exercise:
- Flexibility and range of motion
- Cardio vascular
- Strength training
- Endurance

Being flexible and having full range of motion of your body is important and beautiful. Would you drive a car that the steering wheel was stuck at a maximum range of fifteen degrees? Why live in a body with limited movement? Stretch, do yoga, do something. Joints, bones, ligaments, and tendons all benefit. Part of long life is healthy life.

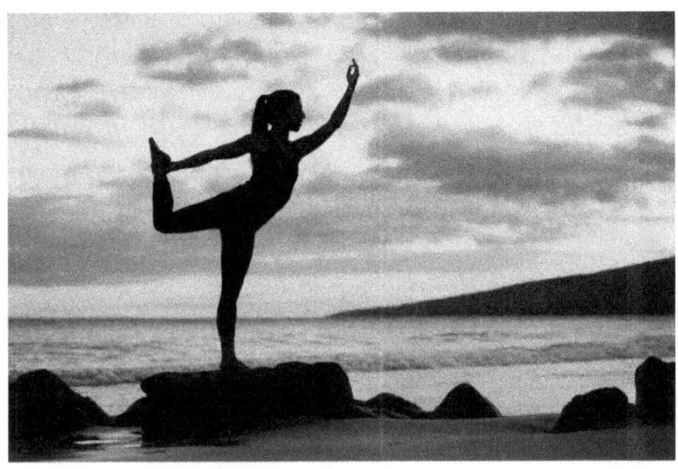

Cardio vascular is probably the most important, because this is how you exercise the heart and brain. Your vasculature is a smooth muscle network. Exercise it. All the little capillaries in the brain benefit from twenty to forty minutes of accelerated pumping a day.

Strength training builds muscles. Muscles are beautiful, so there is the social aspect. Muscles, same as fat, affects your endocrine system. Healthy people have muscle tone, youth and health from an earned physique. Once you are at the level of your choosing, it only takes a few days per week to maintain.

Endurance is the ability to continue for a certain amount of time, like hiking all day or running nonstop for miles. This is based on personal preference and needs.

If you can get your heart rate up to your target rate for twenty minutes and do that three days per week, you are at the most basic level.

There are plenty of books and programs out there. Just do it. Make it a part of your lifestyle. It takes six months to teach your body what the new normal is. First find your fitness level. Second, maintain that level for six months. Third, adopt that new lifestyle as the new you, as your new normal.

The first six pillars will give you a long and healthy life. I believe one hundred and twenty years is possible with just the first six pillars. Giving your body the nutrients it needs to maintain and heal itself, regular exercise, reducing the pathways of accelerated aging, slowing down the biological clock, and keeping yourself in top form for as long as possible is how you will achieve this.

New medical breakthroughs will shatter the glass ceiling of the human life span. 150, 300, and 1000 years will all be in reach given enough time.

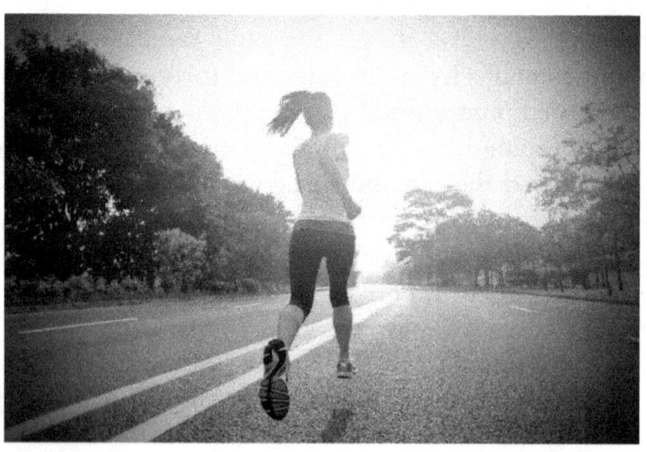

Pillar Seven
Regenerative Medicine

As organs wear out or become diseased, it becomes necessary to replace them. Currently organ transplants have two major problems, availability and compatibility. Currently, to get a transplant, you must wait for another human to die. Not the best moral philosophy. In 1968, the Harvard protocol redefined death to be, "doctor defined brain death." Thirteen men opened the door to a new source of organs; beating heart cadavers. Organ transplants is a twenty billion dollar a year industry. The only ones that can't benefit from it monetarily are the donor's families for ethical reasons.

The study of locked in syndrome and other levels of consciousness have shown that when people are assumed to be brain dead, sometimes that is simply not true. People that know nothing about the transplant industry or the controversy over the process of death are asked to sign the paperwork for a loved one that just died. Guilted into saving some stranger without all the facts or knowledge, but still, there are not enough organs to go around. People die

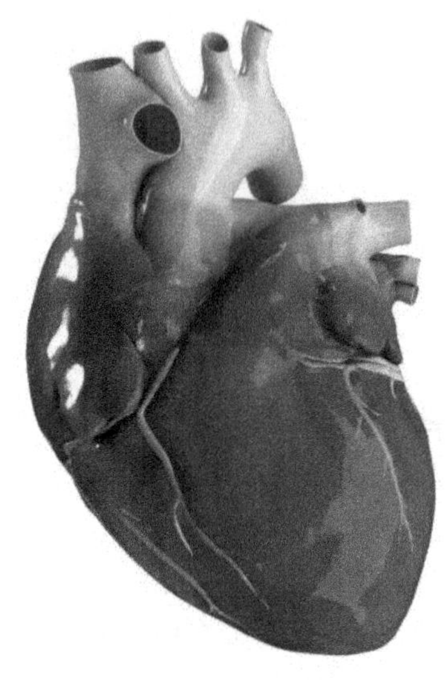

every day from lack of a transplant.

Some poor souls never get to be on the list in the first place. They do not qualify.

Transplanting another person's organs into your body carries the risk of rejection. I was surprised to find out the immunosuppressive drugs for transplant recipients are a billion dollar per year industry. I was also surprised to learn that the toxic nature of immuno-suppressive drugs makes living past ten years very rare. A weakened immune system is another side effect. We need a strong immune system to live a long time. Transplants do not fit the dramatically extended life model.

Science is giving us far better ways. Regenerative medicines will come in three forms. All of which will use your own cells, your own DNA; therefore, eliminating rejection. Your own cells will be harvested from you, grown in a lab to be the exact kind of tissue needed. We will discuss this in the pillar on stem cells.

First, grow an organ by seeding your cells on a protein scaffolding, a protein matrix that will guide growth in a 3D environment, with the right growth factors. A human trachea and bladder have already been grown in this fashion. Technological advances are being made to grow a human heart. The organ would then be transplanted. No waiting for a donor or worrying about rejection. Because no immuno-suppressive drugs are needed, there will be no long-term toxicity. Theoretically, all organs but the brain could be replaced this way.

Second, construct the organ with a 3D bio printer. The protein scaffolding and progenitor cells would be printed together, given nutrients, and the cells given time to take root. The new organ would then be transplanted. No donor, no rejection because it is your own cells. A breakthrough was made in 2014. The vasculature is printed with a gel inside to hold its shape. This temperature dependent gel is then drained out and a nutrient solution pumped through to finish the process. Before, printing depth in the tissue was impossible because the vasculature kept collapsing. Now, it can hold its shape while the cells

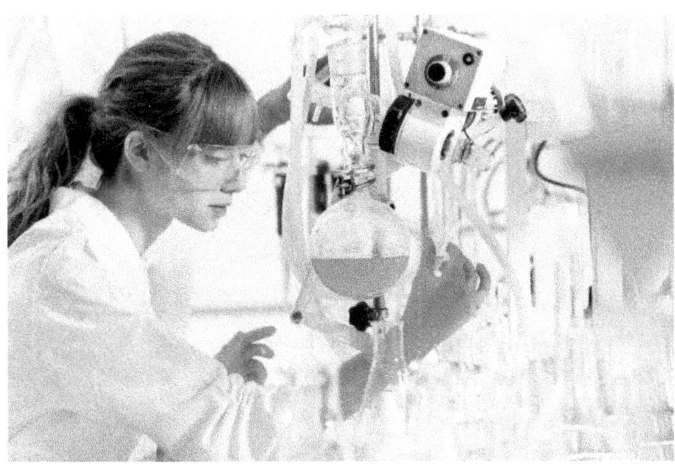

take root. At some point in the future, it may be as simple as unfreezing some of your cells from your "cell bank account" and printing you a new organ. People of the future will rarely die from a failed organ.

Third, direct stem cell injection. The organ would be rebuilt in vivo (in the body). In 2008, a doctor in Brazil injected bone marrow stem cells into a man's heart, directly into the damaged myocardium. The patient went from ashen grey, with a few months to live, to healthy and able to run on the beach.

Direct injection of stem cells and progenitor cells can rejuvenate worn out or diseased organs. The future is bright for organ replacement and regenerative medicine. The transplant industry should embrace this instead of clinging to donors. No rejection means no immunosuppressive drugs. Good for patients. Good for the immune system. Good for a long life.

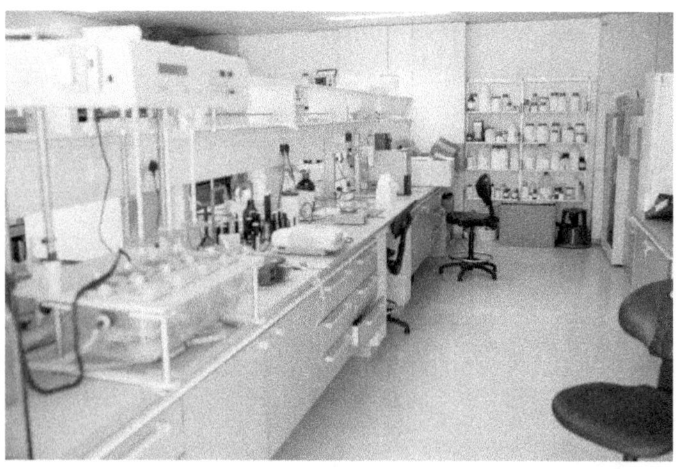

Pillar Eight
Hypothermic Protocol

Each of us needs to rethink what is our definition of death. Does no heartbeat, no breath, and no brain activity really mean death? People are brought back to life after clinical death all the time. Perhaps we should not think of death as a moment in time, but a process. People have drowned in cold water and been clinically dead for over forty-five minutes and brought back to life. In Japan, a woman was brought back after five hours of clinical death.

Brain surgeons will stop their patients heart with cold and preform brain surgery without the heart beating, clinically dead, for up to thirty minutes.

The secret is the cold. Cell death because of oxygen deprivation is a process. The colder the temperature, the slower the biochemical reactions. Brownian motion or the molecular storm speeds up as the temperature rises and slows down as the temperature decreases. It is an established fact that someone can be brought back to life after forty-five minutes of clinical death just because their body was chilled. This should give us pause. What do we really know about death?

Postresuscitation disease is when someone is brought back to life only to die again or suffer brain damage. When we pull someone back across the vail of death, there are a cascade of cellular responses to consider. Cells that have been deprived of oxygen, only to have the hand of death stayed, are not in the clear.

Death is a traumatic event. When the body is brought back to life, the body experiences system wide inflammation, a powerful immune response, and other cellular processes that are poorly understood. Inflammation and immune responses is how the body deals with trauma. The body's response is often so powerful that it kills or damages the brain. This is post resuscitation disease.

The solution is the hypothermic protocol. When someone is brought back to life, induce a medical coma, administer a cocktail of anti-inflammatory and immunosuppressants, and reduce the body's temperature to 89.5 degrees. If we can spread the shock over three days instead of a few hours, the brain can heal on its own. Cold temperatures slow down biochemical reactions. The

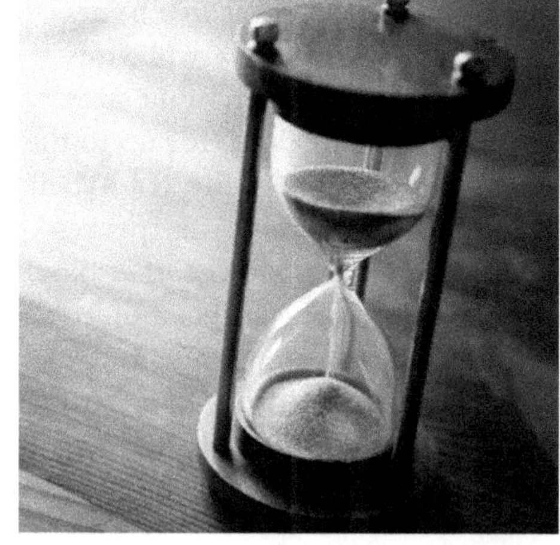

brain must be monitored for swelling. Many people have died because of brain swelling crushing the brain stem. If necessary, use trephining or making a burr hole in the skull to relieve pressure. The swelling will go down if giving enough time.

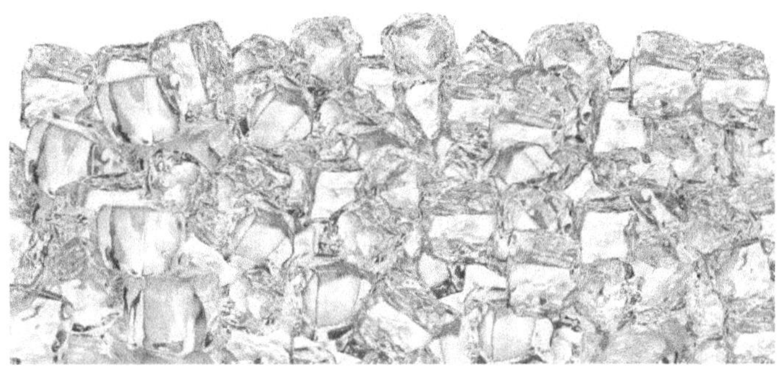

People with head trauma or people that have bled out and died will benefit from the hypothermic protocol. The time needed to replace hearts, fix brain vasculature, stop bleeding et cetera, can be gained by simply cooling the body. There are also extra copular oxygenation machines (ECOM) that can stand in for heart and lungs to pump blood and keep the body oxygenated. Some hospitals use these treatments while others don't. When they tell you that they "did all we could," what does this really mean? If your loved one did not receive forty-five minutes on an ECOM and when they were brought back to life given the hypothermic protocol, well they did not do all they could.

If someone bleeds out or has severe head trauma; cool the body, fix the problem and put them on an ECOM. By cooling the brain, we have additional hours. By placing the patient on an ECOM we have additional days.

The doctor that saved the congress woman who had been shot in the face, used the hypothermic protocol. He commented at a conference that head trauma survival went from two percent to eighty-seven percent with the hypothermic protocol.

I believe that there will come a day when first responders will cool people down on site. People that have had a heart attack, stroke, blood loss, head trauma, et cetera and are pronounced clinically dead and did not respond to CPR will be cooled to 89.5°. At the hospital, they will be put on a ECOM, blood will be transferred, drugs administered, and patients will be stabilized whether their hearts are beating or not. The heart can be replaced with a regenerated one.

There will be a new definition of, "we have done all we can." Death will be understood as a process. A process that can be reversed.

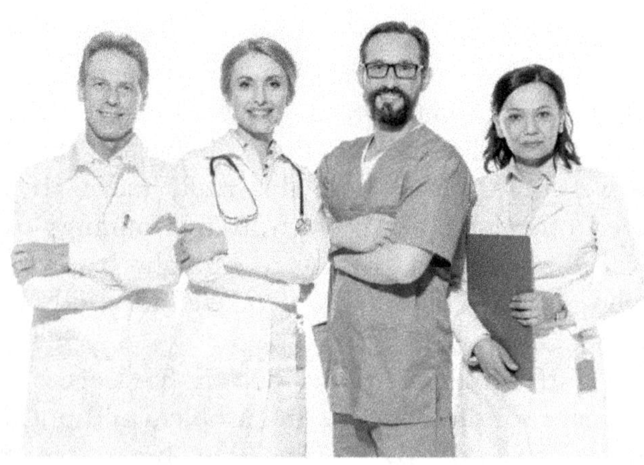

Pillar Nine
Artificial Implants and Nanotechnology

This is truly a remarkable field. Many new industries will be born in the coming years. Many breakthroughs have already been made. When they will be available for the general public is another story. Computer chips implanted on top of the motor cortex have already been used to control robotic arms. Prosthetics that are wired directly in to our nervous system is on the horizon. Artificial organs are already in use. With time, these will be refined. I would imagine in time, replacement arms, legs, kidneys, and hearts will be widely available. As well as, automatic hormone pumps and drug implants.

Medical nanobots are already on the drawing board. We can already make computer chips smaller than the wavelength of light. Nanobots smaller then cells are possible. Immune nanobots to help find and destroy pathogens. Oxygen carrying nanobots to supplement our red blood cells. If someone's lungs were damaged, they could be injected with oxygen carrying life savers. You could also scuba dive without an air tank. A half an hour of oxygen from a single injection. Cancer could be targeted with Nano surgeons. Blood clots would automatically be fixed before you even knew you had a problem. The entire vasculature would be patrolled and maintained by specialized nanobots. The vasculature is a major weakness as we age - strokes, heart disease, thrombotic clots, embolism, and atherosclerosis - nanobots could and some day will maintain these super highways of life.

I would imagine in the future, we will access our computers with our thoughts, and we will be able to download new skill sets and new experiences. Our health will be maintained by an army of nanobots complementing our immune system, inspecting every nanometer of our vasculature, with emergency oxygen and drugs stored away, ready for immediate use. Of course, we would be actively monitored so anything out of the ordinary would be flagged. In an emergency, help would be automatically summoned.

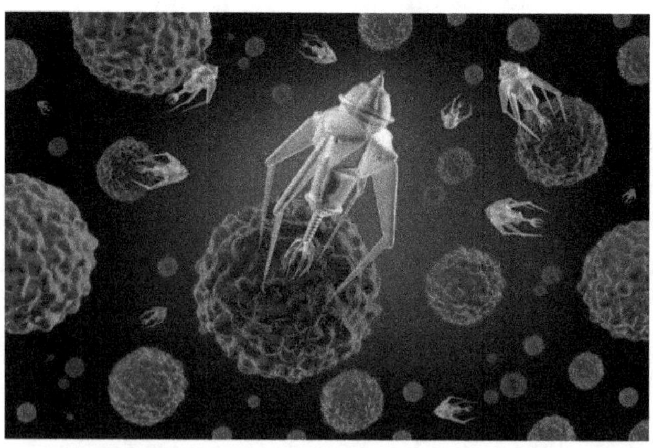

Pillar Ten
Genomics, Gene Therapy, and Gene Expression

Understanding our three billion base pairs of DNA is very different then knowing the three billion A, G, C, & Ts. As we learn how and why genes are expressed and repressed, we will learn about ourselves. Each cell has a complete set of our DNA, yet it is obvious that cells are very different. How our genes are expressed determines the cell type. Lots of our genes are dormant, only to become active in our children.

Four DNA bases, code for twenty amino acids. These amino acids make all the various proteins that make us human. What

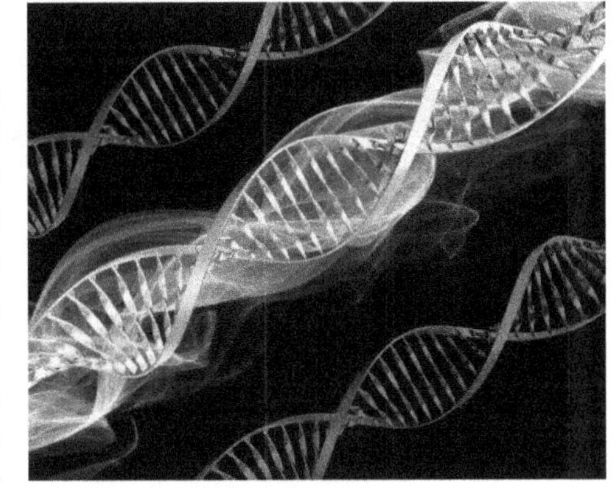

makes oak trees, bacteria, fish, birds, cats, and dogs? DNA. DNA is the code for all life on this planet. How genes are expressed and work together, makes what living things are. Understanding our own 23,000+ or - human genes and how they work together, will make us better, healthier people. We will be able to cure genetic disorders with horizontal gene transfer (HGT).

We need not inherit genes from mom and dad to have access to these genes in the future. Obesity, baldness, propensity for disease, and mutations in the P53, BRCA 1 & 2, APOE, et cetera, could all be treated. Clustered Regularly Interspaced Short Palindromic Repeat (CRISPR) technology promises to do just that.

Understanding and controlling how our genes are expressed, along with the ability to add needed genes, will change human life. Some believe a gene may carry a switch that could extend our lifespan. Just like the gene that was found in C. elegans, that dramatically extended its lifespan.

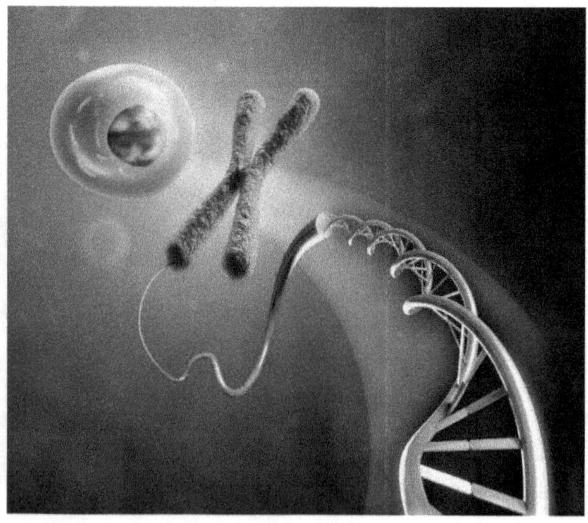

There is no doubt that genes and gene expression affect aging and health. Future babies may be given an extra chromosome at the one cell stage. This twenty-forth chromosome set would be packed will all kinds of dormant genes that could be activated with an activator. You could take a pill and change your hair from blonde to red or a million other useful genetic tweaks awaiting selective activation to cure disease and help us adapt to new environments.

Pillar Eleven
Stem Cells

The miracle of life: a single cell can grow into a human, all the bone, brain, and blood cells and all the muscles, organs, and ligaments. Ten trillion cells and the correct way for them to grow in four-dimensional space. Remarkable. A forest of trees is in the dreams of a single acorn.

A stem cell can turn into any other cell. But the problem is, stem cells have their own DNA. We need stem cells with our own DNA. If when we were an eight-cell mass of undifferentiated cells, a benevolent doctor could swipe one of the cells and keep it frozen for our future self, we would be able to grow an army of our own embryonic stem cells for reseeding our organs at a later date. Identical twins are when the un-differentiated cell ball divides, so it is obvious

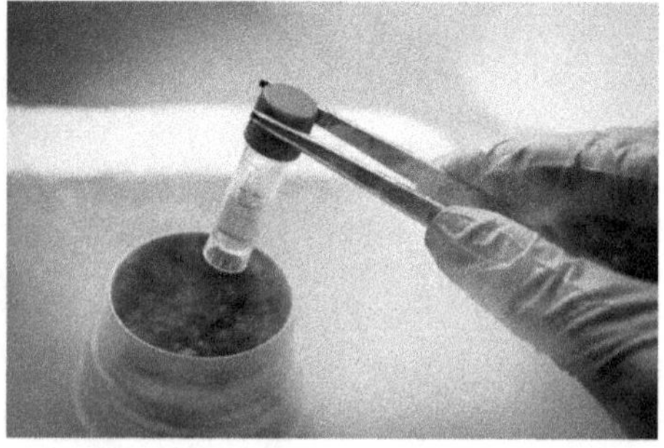

appropriating a single stem cell would not harm our growth.

For those of us without parents with such forethought, there is still hope. We can convince an adult cell to revert back to its stem cell days. Scientists have already made stem cell like cells.

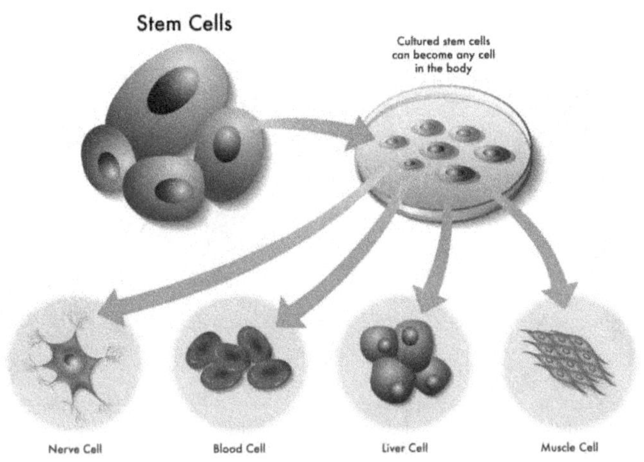

The future will go something like this: we would scratch the inside of your cheek, or perhaps draw some blood, your cells would be isolated, and grown in a nutrient rich solution, RNA vectors and growth factors would be added to revert the cell back to an earlier time, back to an undifferentiated cell, back to a pluri-potent stem cell. As good as we can get to an embryonic stem cell with our own DNA, no embryo needed.

Telomerase would be added to lengthen the telomeres. The cells that mutated or did not transform perfectly would be discarded. This is also the time horizontal gene transfers would be done, if needed. To correct anything that needed correcting. The cells are in the lab and we have easy non-invasive access. We would then grow billions of pristine stem cells. Some would be frozen for future use, and others would be given growth factors to become the cell types that we need. Stem cells and progenitor cells for organ regeneration and cell reseeding would be created.

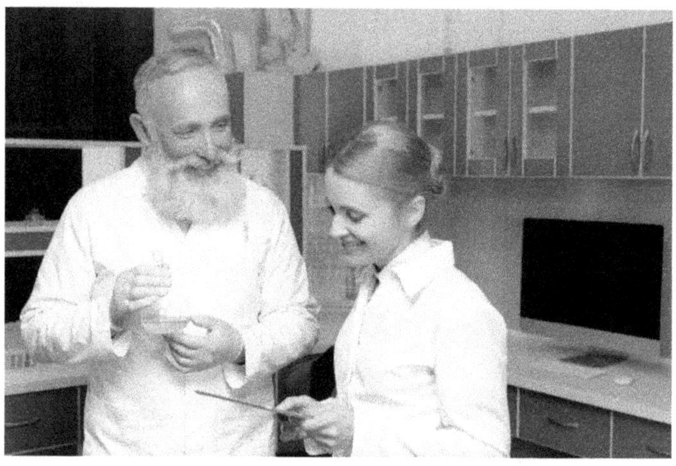

There has been a lot of progress in stem cell research in the last fifteen years. Sadly, because of the open hostility of the US government in the 2000s, other countries have advanced in an industry that America should be leading the world in.

Stem cells will give us the biggest return on our investment when it comes to extending the human life span with stem cell reseeding. Mainstream medicine rejects that aging is a disease because the government does not consider aging to be a disease.

People live too long already in a welfare society, and if the government starts cutting checks at sixty-five, what will happen if people started to live to 150? A nanny state is not compatible with dramatically extended life spans. When the government promises to give you a check until the day you die, they will want you to die sooner rather than later. Once we separate the biological age from the calendar age, new laws could address this.

Life expectancy in the nineteen hundreds was forty-nine. Now, it is in the late seventies. When social security was instituted in 1937, folks were not living that long. Long life equals crisis in the cradle to grave nanny state. It is sad that politics is getting in the way of the greatest revolution the world has ever seen: radical life extension and life spans in the upper one hundreds.

Pillar Twelve
Immunosenescence

Immunosenescence is the "natural" result of the immune system with old age. Immune cells get old and dysfunctional, but won't die and be replaced. They just keep hanging around useless.

The reason that old people are more susceptible to infections is because their immune system is weakened. When a large part of your immune system is senescent, your immune system is compromised.

After a cell has outlived its useful life it goes into apoptosis, or cell suicide. A new cell then takes its place. The immune system is unique in the fact it has "memory." The immune system can remember past pathogens. This means there are long lived

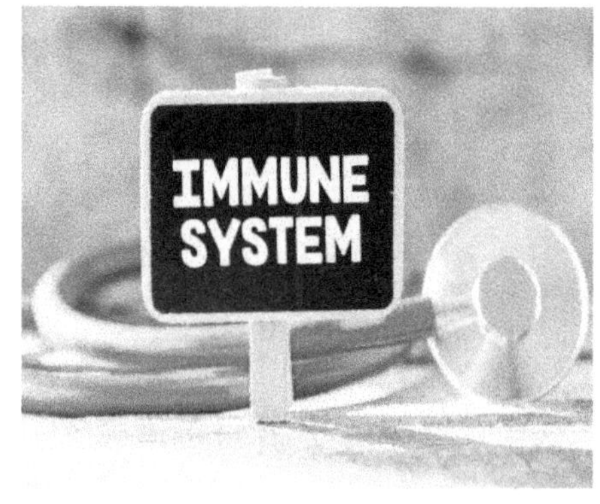

immune cells waiting to recognize a specific threat. Over time these cells lose their ability, become senescent, and are still on the payroll.

Imagine you trained elite warriors to combat invaders. First, they identified the threat. Once they had the codes to the shield, so to speak, your warriors multiplied and then neutralized the invaders. Once the pathogen is eradicated the additional immune cells are no longer needed and go into apoptosis. A remnant will remain that can recognize this threat if it ever invades the body again. All vaccinations are based on this principal. The immune system remembers and can easily destroy those invaders that it recognizes.

Now imagine, over the years of a long life, these immune cells got old and could no longer perform their duties but still made up a part of the immune system's budget. Collecting a pension but no longer able to fight. The immune system command thought it was paying for elite warrior specialists, when in reality it was paying for bingo players. With

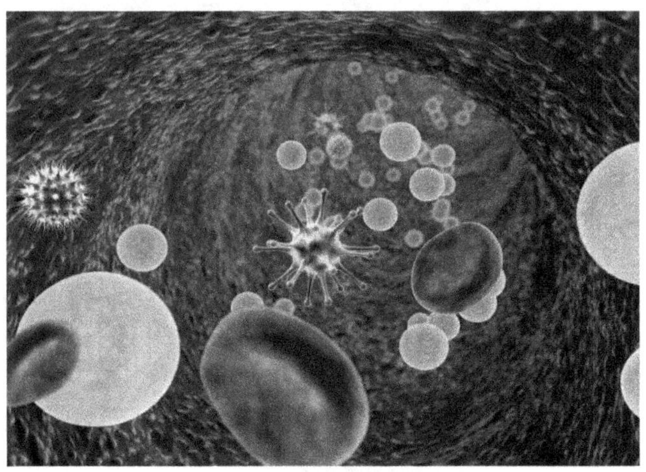

time, the immune system has, in part, become senile.

Your red blood cells are replaced every three months. The bone marrow can crank out billions of white blood cells if needed. A robust immune system is needed for a long life. The stem cells in you bone marrow that make red and white blood cells can be replaced. Bone marrow transplants are common. Reseeding your bone marrow with your own lab-grown stem cells is an obvious solution once your bone marrow stem cells have reached the Hayflick Limit.

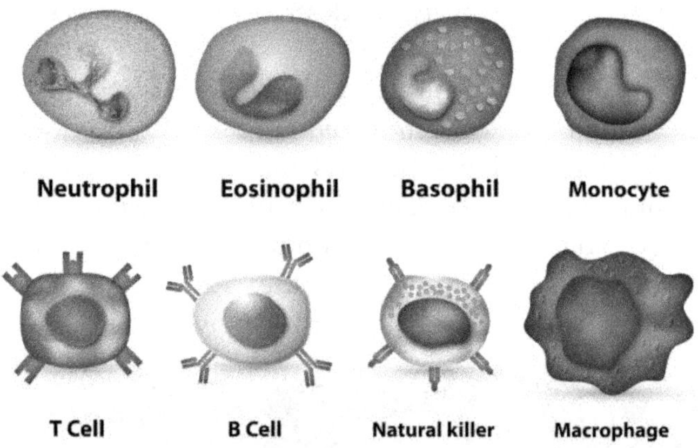

People that have immunosenescence often have robust blood cell factories in their bones. The problem is not producing immune cells but triggering the need to produce immune cells.

The solution is to purge the senescent immune cells which will in turn trigger their replacement. Drugs are being developed that target the toxic markers of senescent cells. Four-day water fasts purge senescent immune cells. Nanobots could be programed to destroy senescent immune cells. Quercetin has been shown to help as well.

Purging senescent immune cells and stem cell reseeding should give us a robust immune system into extreme old age. Old age will be seen as a mark of wisdom and experience. Now old age is the slow, visible onset of death. Hundred and fifty-year olds will have the immune systems of thirty-year olds.

Right now, five of the top twelve killers of the ninety to one hundred year old age bracket, is connected with a poor immune system. Anytime you hear that an elderly person died of an infection, they really died of immunosenescence. A strong immune system is a pillar of a long life.

Pillar Thirteen
General Senescence

Save for your brain and heart cells, all of your cells are replaced on a regular timetable. Each tissue has its own cycle. Intestinal cells every 5-7 days. Bone cells every 5-7 years. Muscle cells as needed. Blood cells every three months. The liver regenerates, you can even cut chunks out of your liver, and it will regrow. Each tissue has its own time table for replacement. The disease of aging affects this cycle.

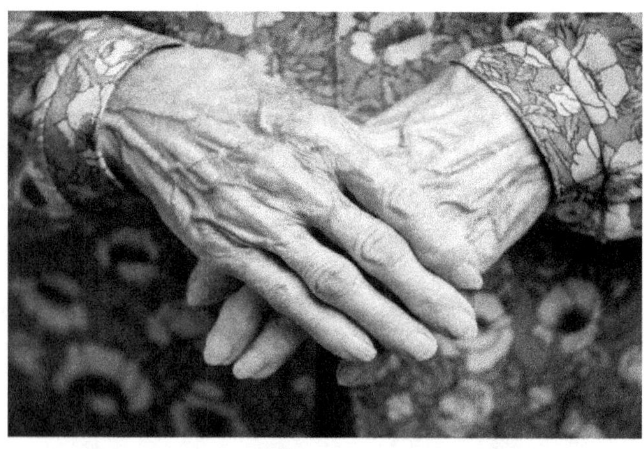

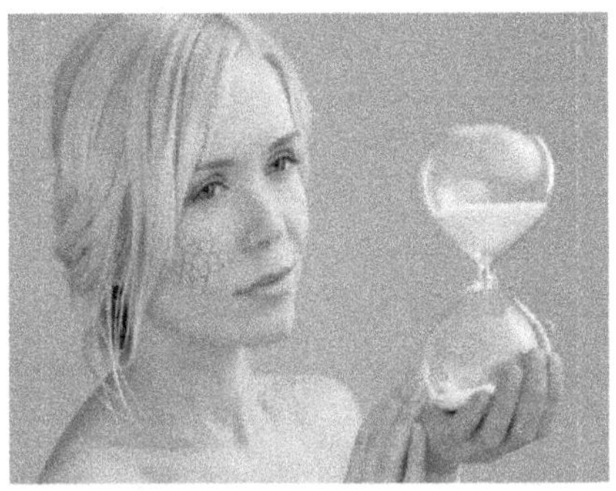

With time, some cells degenerate into senescent cells. Poorly functioning or dysfunctioning cells that just hang around. These zombie cells create inflammation, misshaped proteins, free radicals and even sometimes results in cancer.

Cells have mechanisms to repair themselves and to go into apoptosis (cell suicide) if they cannot make themselves whole again. Senescence is a failure in engaging in apoptosis. The immune system can tag faulty and precancerous cells for destruction. So immunosenescence affects general senescence. The accumulation of senescent cells is a biological marker of old age.

Drugs are being developed that target senescent cells. There are promising studies already done with mice. To take a pill or hook up an IV to purge your senescent cells every five years, would be ideal. Everyone over thirty has some senescent cells, but old people have far more. Once a threshold has been reached, the zombie cells effect on the quality of your life becomes noticeable. I would imagine in the future, treatments to purge senescent cells would begin at forty-five years of age.

As our stem cells reach their Hayflick Limit, the body is not so quick to destroy old cells. Poorly functioning senescent cells, at this point, help hold together a poorly functioning body. Washing away all the senescent cells in a hundred-year-old body could have disastrous consequences. When that's all you have got and the stem cells are few and far between, senescent cells perform a function. Stem cell seeding is of course the solution to this. The 23 pillars all work together.

Taking care of yourself by applying the first six pillars, will reduce the burn rate of your cells. A toxic lifestyle requires accelerated cell replacement. Teens and twentysomethings do not realize the damage they are doing, because it is hidden by cell replacement. Always consider the burn rate that you are going through healthy cells. The Hayflick Limit gives us about forty to fifty divisions of our stem cells. Beyond this we would need stem cell reseeding with cells that have had their telomeres repaired and cell organelles regenerated. This is all possible with future technology.

Four-day water fasts and Quercetin can help purge senescent cells until a drug is available or nanobots are invented, but we must do all we can to reduce the burn rate of our core stem cells.

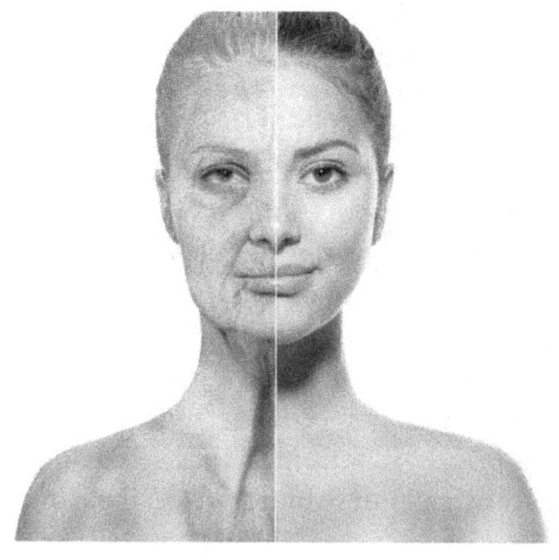

Pillar Fourteen
Cell Loss and Atrophy

Cell loss is a biological marker of aging. As our stem cells decrease, we make do with less muscles and tissues of all kinds. Cell loss is system wide and slow. Cell loss and atrophy is a visible marker of age. Cell loss is accepted as a natural course of aging. The solution is stem cell reseeding. Until medical advancements are made, the best we can do is to reduce our stem cell burn rate. If we take care of ourselves, by applying the first six pillars, we should be able to make it to a hundred and twenty which is close to the upper limit for the human lifespan at present.

When cell loss reaches a tipping point and body functions can no longer be maintained, this is a visible sign of aging. This happens at different rates for different people based on lifestyle and genetics.

Pillar Fifteen
Telomeres

Telomeres are the end caps that hold DNA together and get shorter with each cell division. The Hayflick Limit is when the telomere gets so short that the cell can't function. Normally at this point the cell will go into apoptosis. With old age and other disorders, the cell may turn senescent.

Short telomeres for cells that are going to sluff off and die (skin, intestinal cells, et cetera) is not

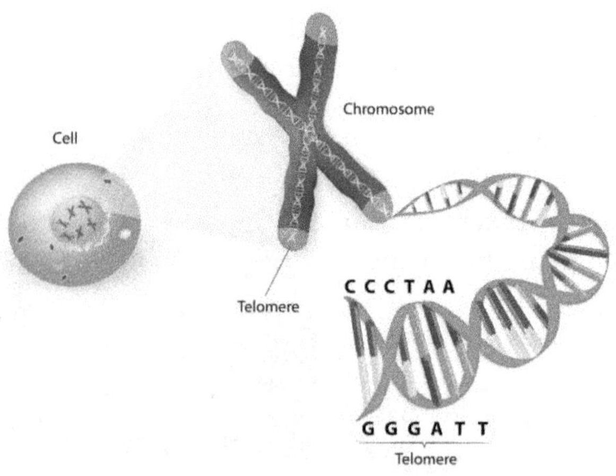

a problem. Cells that are about to be replaced anyway have no need for robust telomeres. Stem cells and progenitor cells do. Short telomeres are a biological yard stick for aging. When we say biological age, telomere length is a major factor.

Telomerase is an enzyme that lengthens telomeres but can also cause cancer. One of the things that most cancers need to grow is to activate the telomerase gene. The solution is to grow our billions of stem cells in a lab and discard the precancerous and mutated cells. Cancer is not the only thing that can lengthen telomeres. Germ cells (sperm and egg) lengthen the telomeres as a matter of course. Every once in a while, a clone will have lengthened telomeres too.

Nature has shown that telomeres can be lengthened. It is just a matter of working out the details. Stem cell reseeding depends on this. I will note, if you took and froze some cells from when you were a baby, you would have a stem cell pool with long telomeres. Even cryobanking stem cells from when you are forty years old, your telomeres will be far longer than when your ninety years old.

It is recommended to save some of your stem cells as soon as it is financially feasible. The procedure is simple; fat is sucked out of your abdomen, the stem cells are separated with a centrifuge, and the stem cells are then put in liquid nitrogen for long-term storage, cryobanking.

Some supplements and drugs have shown promise. There is a company that charges over $50,000 for a protocol that says it can help with lengthening your telomeres. Resveratrol also has shown some promise. There may be a day in the future where it becomes common to lengthen telomeres periodically. This biological clock can and will be stopped or slowed down and rewound.

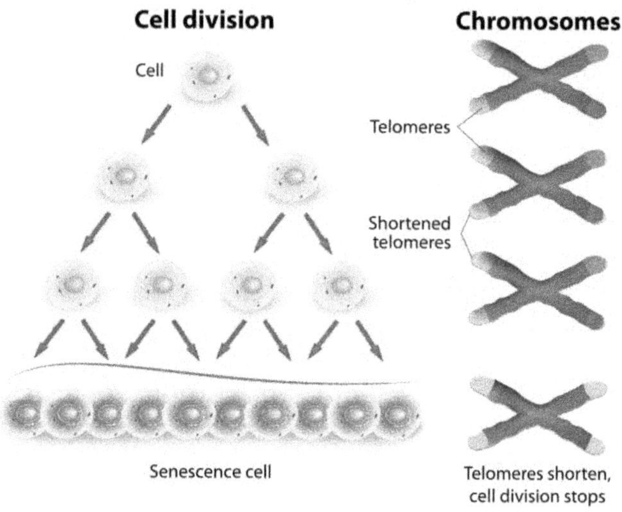

Pillar Sixteen
Mitochondria Mutations

Mitochondria are the power plants of the cells. Mitochondria are self-replicating organelles that are in the cytoplasm of every cell in your body. The oxygen we breath is used to fuel our mitochondria. Mitochondria makes ADP, the energy currency of the cell.

Mitochondria juggle electrons and transport protons to make ADP out of sugars and fats. About every two weeks the hundreds of mitochondria per cell are replaced. Mitochondria have their own DNA, and it is passed down from mother to baby, unlike the 23 chromosomes from mom and dad that make up the DNA in the cell nucleus.

Mitochondria have their own DNA and replicate on their own time table. The old mitochondria are recycled by our lysosomes. All of our energy needs come from these little power plants. Without ADP, our cells would die quickly. We cannot pick up a cup of coffee or think a thought without ADP. Healthy mitochondria are beyond important to life; they produce the energy of life. Any discussion

of radical life extension would be incomplete without
an analysis of mitochondria.

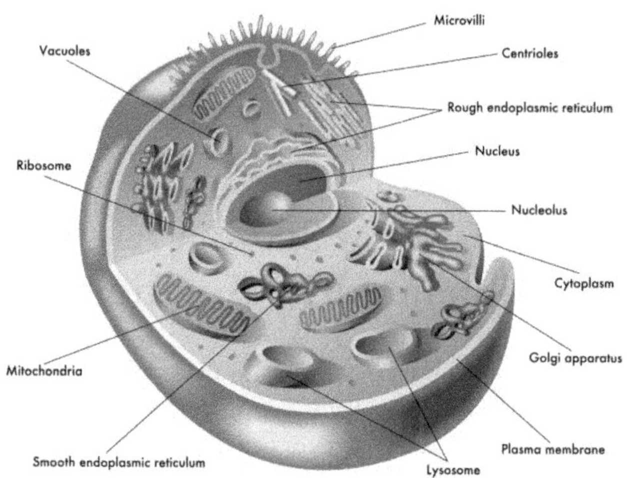

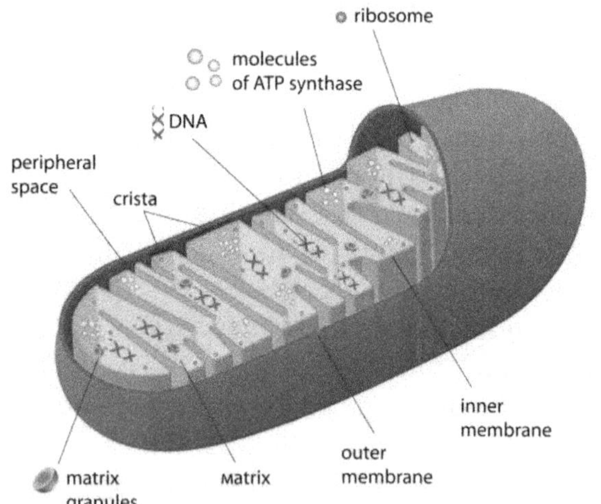

Mitochondrion

Mitochondria mutations cause cells to fail. Solutions are many. Gene therapy, nanobots to inject fresh mitochondria, and virus vectors with the DNA code to build fresh mitochondria all show promise. There are supplements like CoQ10 that help support healthy mitochondria as well.

We would make sure as we develop stem cell reseeding that the new cells would have robust mitochondria. It would be fairly easy to inject robust mitochondria into the cytoplasm of your stem cell lines. Already folks with congenital defects in their mitochondria can get "donor" mitochondria. The newspapers called it, "I have two mommies," one from the 23 chromosomes from the mother's egg, and one from the mitochondrial DNA in organelles of the donners cytoplasm. Hundreds of mitochondria float in each of our cells. I suspect the number is considerably higher in a human egg cell.

Cells with faulty mitochondria normally die or turn senescent. We would need to purge the senescent cells, but the long lived brain and heart cells are a different deal and will require repair in the body. The heart is an organ that could be replaced if necessary but not the brain. We have neurons in our brain that have been with us from when we were in our mother's womb. Brain mitochondria must be fixed in the brain. Fixing the mitochondria in the rest of the body will be easy compared to this. Stem cell reseeding is the obvious choice for every cell in the body, save for our neurons in the neocortex. We could reseed the hippocampus because it deals in short term memories. We must tread carefully when working on parts of the brain that makes us who we are.

Pillar Seventeen
Advanced Glycation End Products (AGEs) and Protein Crosslinks

When a sugar molecule binds to a functional protein through a process known as glycation, that protein is rendered dysfunctional and undergoes further structural rearrangements. The end result is advanced glycation end products, or AGEs. This can affect any tissue where blood goes. In others words, the entire extracellular matrix. AGEs accumulate in the brain, kidneys, skin, arteries, et cetera as we get older. One of the causes of wrinkles on your skin is from AGEs. When the protein collagen binds with a sugar molecule and glycates, it goes from tough and flexible to brittle and stiff. Just pinch the cheeks of a child and then pinch the cheek of eighty-year old, and see the difference in flexibility and resiliency. AGEs are a major factor. Properly shaped collagen is needed for a youthful face as well as a youthful brain and body.

Protein crosslinks is just what it sounds like:

proteins that have linked or become tangled together and become dysfunctional. Proteins are manufactured by cells to preform specific functions. A misshapen or crosslinked protein cannot perform its function. A Thanksgiving turkey gives us a good example. A lifetime of crosslinks in a few hours. Think of how soft and supple the turkey's skin is when you first put it in the oven. The heat accelerates the formation of the protein crosslinks.

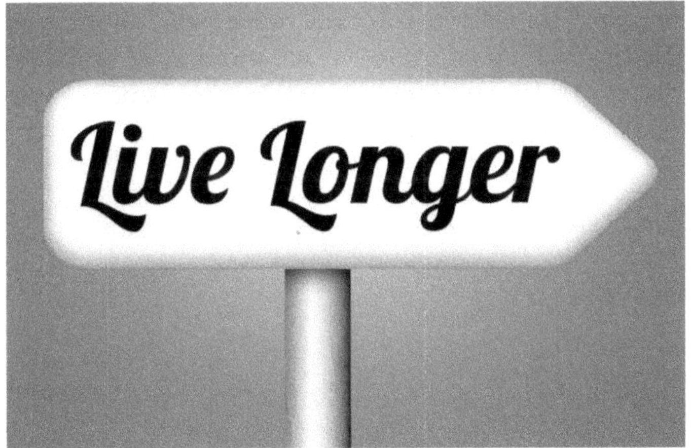

AGEs and protein crosslinks are both biological markers of aging. Over a lifetime they accumulate. They are tangled in your extra cellular matrix. Look at someone's face and you have a good idea of how old they look like inside.

There are other factors to a wrinkled face. Old cells make less proteins in the first place. Senescent cells don't make any useful proteins and spew free radicals. Hyaluronic acid is depleted so skin is not as thick or hydrated. Hyaluronic acid holds a thousand times its weight in water and is needed in your eyes, joints, arteries, as well as your skin. Vitamins like A, E, D and K2 also play a part in healthy skin.

There are drugs in development to breakdown AGEs and protein crosslinks, but they are a long way off. Nanobots may be able to help in the future. The best practice is to slow down the creation of AGEs and protein cross links in the first place. Excess sugar causes glycation. Free radicals, radiation, and toxins cause most of the protein crosslinks. If you practice the first six pillars, you will reduce the amount of AGEs and crosslinks you accumulate in the first place. At least getting you over the hundred-year mark. In time, there will be other treatments.

Pillar Eighteen
Intercellular Junk and Lipofuscin Buildup

Inside each of our cells are organelles called lysosomes. These little organelles go around the cells and clean up the garbage. Lysosomes digest and recycle everything from proteins to old mitochondria. They are like the garbage collectors of your cells.

Over time, lipofuscin builds up in the lysosomes making them inefficient and at some point dysfunctional. Imagine the garbage truck dumping its load at the county landfill. The congealed residue that sticks to the bottom and sides of the inside of the dump truck box is a good comparison to the lipofuscin that sticks to the inside of the lysosomes.

Cells that die and are replaced, are not really a problem for lipofuscin buildup. The long-lived cells are our concern here. When a person dies peacefully in his sleep, when his heart just stops beating, without the pain and struggle of an oxygen deprived heart attack, it is usually caused because of lipofuscin build up. Sometimes, ten percent of the weight of a hundred plus year old heart, is often lipofuscin.

We need to develop a drug that the lysosomes will recognize as trash and clean out of the insides of our cells. This drug would then have a component that cleaned out the lysosomes. Sort of like an intercellular liquid plumber.

Hearts can be regrown and replaced if the lipofuscin cannot be cleaned out of the lysosomes. Stem cell lines would be given fresh lysosomes. Not so with the long-lived cells in our brains. We need to address this problem to expand our lifespan past one hundred and twenty. Like most of the, "Past a hundred and twenty years old problems," the brain is central.

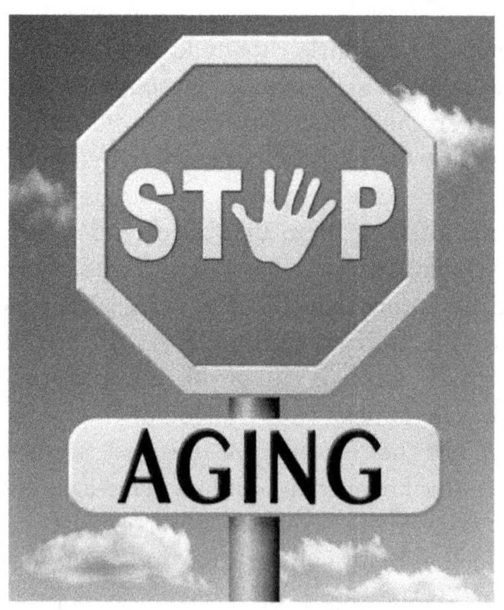

Pillar Nineteen
Extracellular Misshapen Proteins and Extracellular Junk

There are many forms of extracellular misshapen proteins and extracellular junk. Alzheimer's disease and prion disease are two examples.

Alzheimer's disease is the result of a buildup of misshapen proteins known as amyloid beta. Misshapen proteins are the result of cells producing misshapen proteins in the first place or something misshaping them at a later point.

In prion disease, a prion (which is a protein itself) turns other proteins into proteins like itself.

DNA codes for sixty-four codons that tell the RNA how to arrange twenty amino acids. DNA only codes for amino acids and all human proteins are made out of twenty amino acids. Misshapen proteins are a big deal if they get out of hand.

The body has methods for clearing out extracellular junk. Namely the immune system. The immune system normally does not cross the blood brain barrier. The Microglia brain cells act as the brain's immune system.

There was a clinical trial where the microglia were "vaccinated" against the amyloid beta protein. Some people died from brain swelling, others were cured of Alzheimer's. If a disease kills a hundred percent of its victims and the cure kills twenty percent, the FDA will protect you from the dangerous cure.

Alzheimer's disease is the second leading cause of death for people over ninety. The ten to twenty years before you die from Alzheimer's can be worse than death. Alzheimer's is a road block to a long-life span. If you live long enough, you probably will get it. Young people will sometimes get this disease too, if they have a mutation in the APOE gene. There has been a lot of research in this field. Millions are being spent to find a cure for Alzheimer's disease.

All misshapen proteins and extracellular junk must be addressed to dramatically extend our lives. We need a method of cleaning our brains of misshapen proteins and extracellular waste.

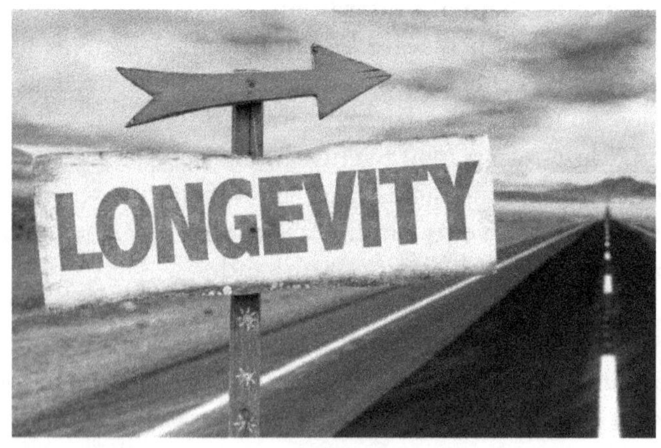

Pillar Twenty
DNA Mutations and Cancer

DNA mutations cause a lot of problems; the most well-known is cancer. With billions of cells dividing, mutations can propagate. Mutations of stem cells and progenitor cells is all we need to concern ourselves with. Business end cells that are working and/or have a limited life, are of no concern to us. For example: if a skin cell has a mutation and is sluffed off, no harm, or in your colon, a mutated cell that is replaced in five days is left in the toilet causing no harm.

Colon cancer and skin cancer is because of a progenitor cell that had a nuclear mutation. Uncontrollable cell division resulting in an eventual metastasis. (Metastasis is where the tumor seeds cancer cells throughout the body.) People don't die of colon cancer and skin cancer, as much as from secondary tumors caused by the primary tumor.

Stem cells and progenitor cells that have a mutation in their DNA can reproduce at a very fast rate and turn in to a tumor.

DNA mutations can happen four ways:

radiation, chemo toxins, viruses, and a breakdown of the cells repair systems. As a cell divides, mutations are found and repaired. If they cannot be repaired the cell goes into apoptosis. Most cancers/cell mutations are repaired, or the cell will commit suicide. It is estimated that 20,000 mutations are fixed in in the human body every day. A normal person living a normal healthy life, does not even know of this battle waged within. If the mutated cell fails to kill itself, the immune system will often recognize it as defective and attack.

For cancer to be successful, it first needs a mutation for runaway cell growth. Second, it must "cloak" itself from the immune system which is easier with a biologically old immune system. Third, it must activate angiogenesis, the formation of new blood vessels. Forth, it must activate the telomerase gene; otherwise, the Hayflick Limit would limit the tumor before it was even noticeable. Cancer is the second largest killer of people right behind diseases of the heart. If you live long enough, you will get cancer.

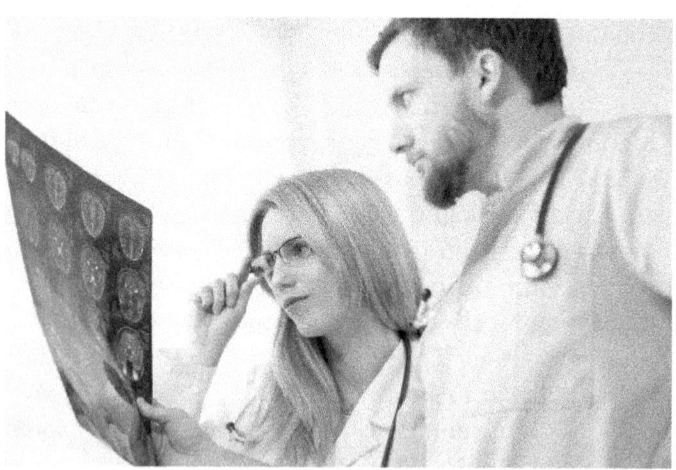

A strong immune system is the best defense. Find out if you have a propensity with genetic testing. Avoid unnecessary radiation, toxins, and viruses, practice the first six pillars, and find cancer with early detection.

Avoid metastasized cancers through early detection. It is far easier to destroy cancer at stage one.

Stem cell research will help us with a cure. Because cancer is a disease of the stem cells. New drugs, immunotherapy, nanobots, fasting therapy, proton therapy, and a healthy lifestyle are the best we have right now. All other DNA mutations are small potatoes compared to cancer but will need to be addressed as we proceed to dramatically extended the human life span.

Pillar Twenty-One
Old Age Brain Diseases

With stem cell reseeding and organ regeneration, the body can be rejuvenated bit by bit or organ by organ. Not so with the brain. The essences of who we are is our brain. We need to fix our neurons without replacing them.

Some brain cell classes could probably be stem cell reseeded, like the supporting brain cells: microglia, astrocytes, and oligo dendrites. Brain regions that do not hold long term memories could also be reseeded, like the dopamine producing cells that fail in Parkinson's disease or the short-term memory cells in the hippocampus.

For neurons of our neocortex, we will have to find a way to rebuild the cells in the

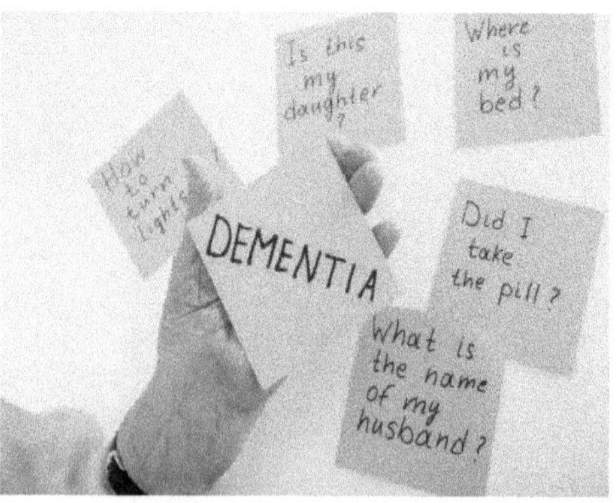

brain by fixing and/or replacing organelles like the mitochondria and lysosomes.

Each brain disease must be analyzed and addressed. A clean and healthy vasculature is the best way to maintain a healthy brain. Practice the first six pillars now, and live long enough to see the breakthroughs that are being researched right now.

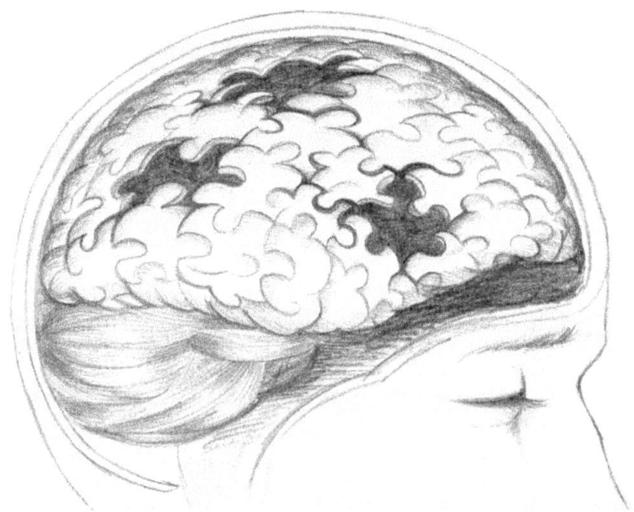

Pillar Twenty-Two
New Diseases and Proactive Research

Malaria, typhus, cholera, smallpox, Spanish flu, the bubonic plague, AIDS, polio, and TB used to kill people by the millions. Life expectancy has doubled over the last two hundred years. Childhood mortality has fallen dramatically. Many history books will tell of families that had seventeen children, only to have two survive.

Modern medicine and antibiotics has changed life as we know it. The quality of life and the length of life have been improved, but with a longer life comes diseases that were not a problem for the short lived. If you are going to die at thirty or forty, is cancer or Alzheimer's a problem for the general population? Old people can now be kept alive longer, sometimes so they can live sickly lives. In the past, the frailties of old age were less of a problem because people often died much younger. People were not kept alive with advanced medical treatments. Some people advocate for a return to a simpler time when people died with dignity. Sometimes when you hear, "die with dignity," it's code for pulling the plug or giving up.

The idea that there are diseases that affect the elderly because they are old is a simple concept. If we cure aging, a lot of the old age diseases will disappear. As we change our biological age, we cut at the root of the aging process.

It is also reasonable to assume that if we start living to a hundred and fifty years on average, we will encounter new diseases that we will have to find cures for. We must always be forever vigilant. Just like we cured childhood mortality going from below fifty percent to the high nineties, we will cure the diseases specific to advanced old age.

I think we should be ever watchful. If we cure what is killing us now and start to live over a hundred and fifty, there is probably new diseases that we can't even imagine waiting for us in the future. We must be always ready and prepared with resources, technology, and skilled minds capable of original thought to aggressively attack the illnesses and diseases of tomorrow.

The one hundred and fifty-year old must expect new challenges in the future.

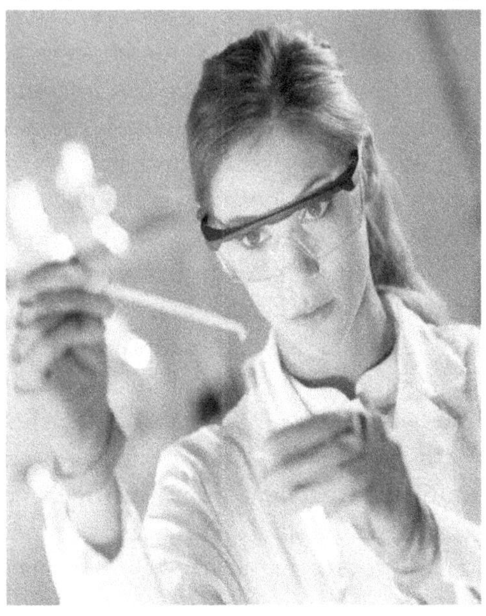

Pillar Twenty-Three
Cryonics Arrangements

Cryonics is hope rooted in logic and science. Death is a process. Cold slows down this process. Liquid nitrogen stops the process. Hence the term "suspended animation." Technology keeps improving. To believe that technology will stop improving is a denial of history. If we judge the future from our past, then technology will continue to improve beyond what we can imagine. There is an old saying, if you ask an elderly respected scientist if something is possible, and he says "yes," he is most likely right. If he answers, "no", he is most likely wrong.

Nature already has fauna that will freeze and come back to life when the temperature rises. A rabbit kidney has been frozen and brought back to a functional state in the lab. C. elegans has been frozen, and when brought back to life, shown to retain its memories in the lab. Sperm, eggs, and embryos are routinely frozen in liquid nitrogen and brought back to life, reanimated. Thousands of people are walking around today that used to be a frozen embryo.

Cryonics is a backup plan to dramatically extend the human life span. If the technology of today cannot fix aging, then the technology of the future can. By slowing the death process to a stop, we can give ourselves the time.

The process of cryonics involves washing out the blood and filling the body with a cryoprotectant solution to avoid crystallization upon freezing. The brain will be in suspended animation until a point in the future where technology will reanimate us and cure aging.

No one can know the promise of future technology. Anyone who would claim what cannot be done in the future is like a cave man sitting around a fire trying to contemplate our modern life. We do not have the resources or context to even make an educated guess. What we can be sure of, is it will be dramatic.

Technology doesn't progress on a linear scale; technology progresses is on an exponential scale.

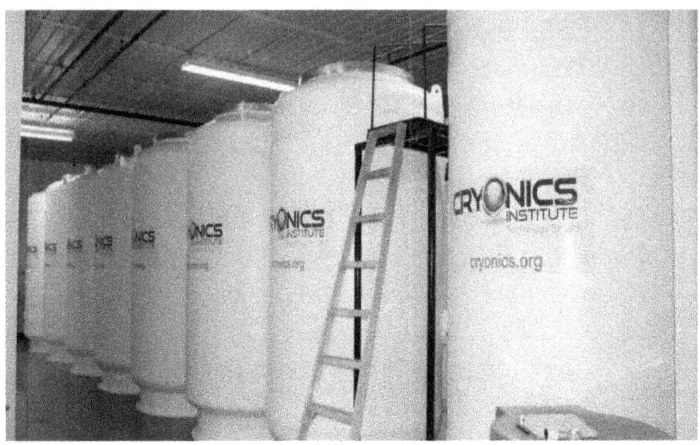

THE 23 PILLARS OF
ESOTERIC GERONTOLOGY

1. Sleep And Recovery
2. Hydration, Detoxification, Inflammation, And Oxidation
3. Diet And Nutrition
4. Nutraceuticals
5. Hormone Balance
6. Exercise
7. Regenerative Medicine
8. Hypothermic Protocol
9. Artificial Implants And Nano Technology
10. Genomics, Gene Therapy, And Gene Expression
11. Stem Cell Colonies And Stem Cell Reseeding
12. Immunosenescence
13. General Senescence
14. Cell Loss And Cell Atrophy
15. Telomeres
16. Mitochondria Mutations
17. Advanced Glycation End Products And Protein Cross Links
18. Intercellular Junk, Lipofuscin Build Up
19. Extra Cellular Junk And Misshapen Proteins
20. DNA Mutations And Cancer
21. Old Age Brain Diseases
22. New Diseases And Proactive Research
23. Cryonics Arrangements

We can understand aging and extend the human life span. Above are the 23 areas of research and focus that will make all the difference. The longer that we can live, the better chance we have that we will live longer. People are living longer than ever before. The human race will cure this most terrible disease that has cursed us through the ages. A disease built into the very fabric of our being, but a disease nonetheless, that just needs a cure. Or in this case, a complex twenty-three pronged attack.

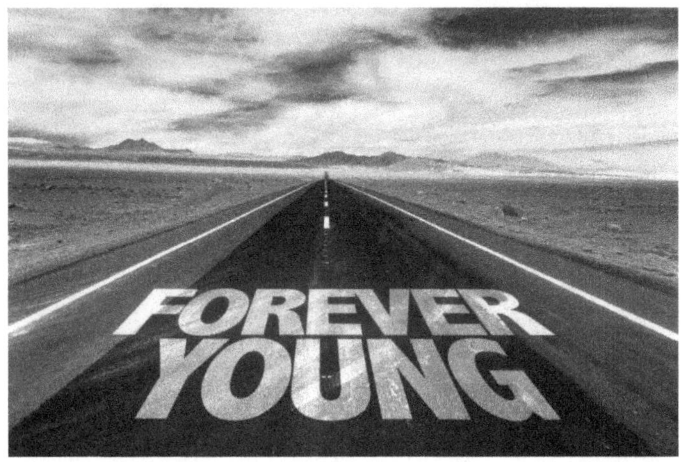

"There is nothing in biology yet found that indicates the inevitability of death. This suggests to me that it is not at all inevitable and that it is only a matter of time before biologists discover what it is that is causing us the trouble and that this terrible universal disease or temporariness of the human's body will be cured."

- Nobel Laureate, Richard Feynman

"Do not go gentle into that good night. Rage, rage against the dying of the light."
- Dylan Thomas

"One more cup of coffee, one more summer day, one more day to explore, learn, and create. One more day to spend time with the ones you love."
-Duke Watrous

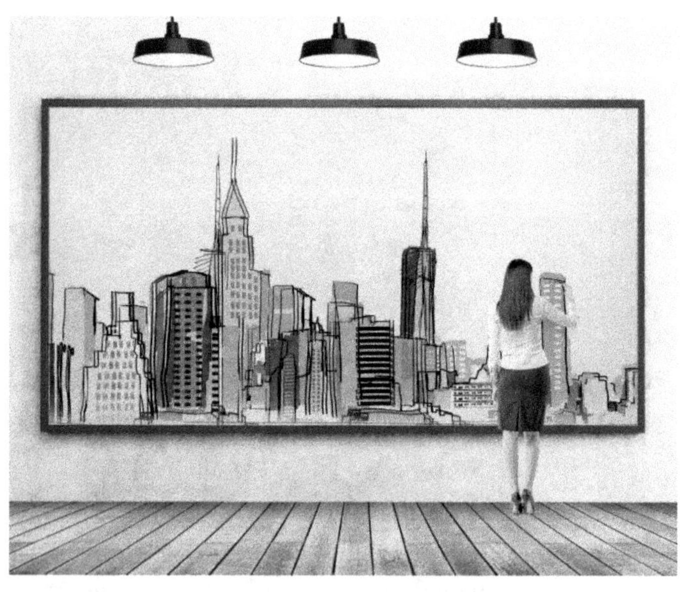

Think About It.

Why would we not what to live longer? Why do we accept death as certain? For the first time in human history, we can describe the aging process at the cellular level. Why would we not do something about it?

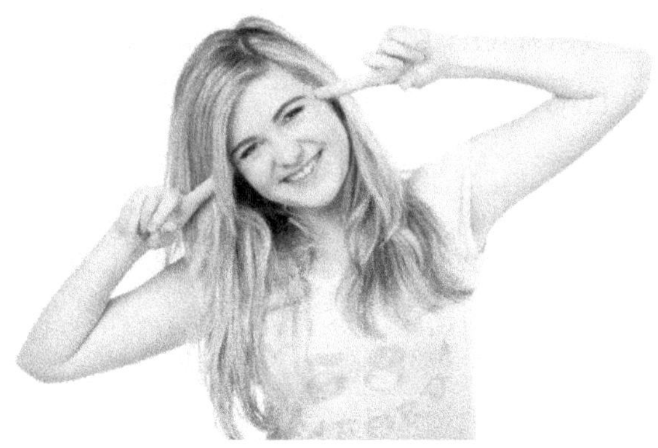

Buy books in bulk and tell the world. This is our generation's moon shot. We must end aging. www.dukewatrous.com

Dear Reader,

I wanted to thank you from the bottom of my heart for reading this little book. This project has become very dear to my heart over the years that I have reflected, pondered, studied the aging process, and what can be done about it. I really hope this book has made you see the world in a new light.

The value of a book is not measured in book sales, but in how words can touch the human heart. I hope you found value in this book. I hope the pages have become dogeared with sentences underlined and paragraphs highlighted. Coffee stains and wear are the mark of a book that is used and loved. Books that sit on the bookshelf in perfect condition do little good beyond decoration.

Nothing can help a book gain traction like personal recommendations from family and trusted friends. Nothing can propel a book forward more than the reviews of those that have actually read the book. I will be grateful for every positive review you take the time to write. Please go to where you bought this book and take the time to write a review. Please post a comment on your social media for your friends and family to see.

Sales of this book benefit the Ashley Watrous Foundation. Thank you again for taking the time to read my book.

Sincerely,

Duke Watrous

The Ashley Watrous Foundation

Every sale of this book helps benefit the Ashley Watrous Foundation. The Ashley Watrous Foundation is dedicated to helping young scientists, inventors, and entrepreneurs through grants, education, and mentorship.

See www.AshleyWatrous.org for a grant application, more information, or to make a donation.

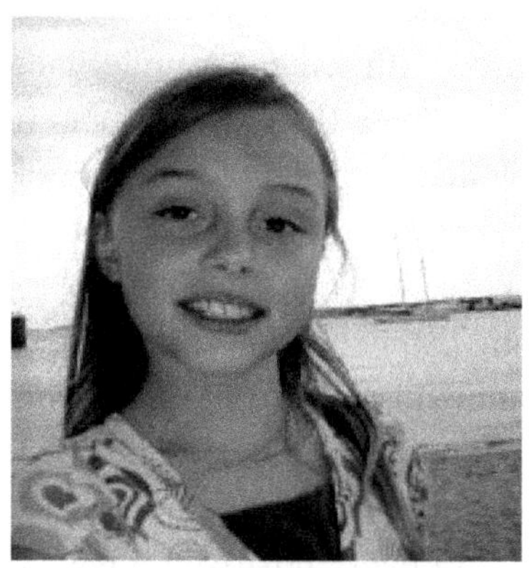

Martha's Vineyard, Summer 2009
Copywrite © 2009 The Author

Ashley was a brilliant, beautiful, and a happy little girl with a sparkling personality. She died on Christmas Eve 2009. A tragic accident at the hands of the man that loved her more than anything, her father. The purpose of this foundation is so she will be remembered and good will be done in her name.

Ashley was a kind and gentle soul. May this foundation reflect her desire to help others and her big heart.

ABOUT THE AUTHOR

I am a libertarian, a patriot, and a firm believer in individual responsibility. I am a father, a son, and a brother. I love my kids more than anything.

In my life, I have been a ranch hand, an amateur vet, a horse trainer, a chicken herder, a fisherman, a river floater, a welder, a mechanic, a gardener, a landscaper, a hunter, a telemarketer, a film coupon book salesman, a phonebook delivery man, a security system salesman, a traveling book salesman, a guardian of my brothers, a crew chief for a magic show, a furniture mover, a parasail boat captain, a house rehabber, a fence builder, a truck driver, a logistical analyst, a small business owner, an entrepreneur, a job creator, a traveler, a board game inventor, and I have four stepped under the hot Texas sun in a prison field squad.

I have been madly in love, and I have experienced profound betrayal. I have been through a bitter divorce, and I have fought for my children within the legal system. I have created wealth and gone bankrupt with the crashing economy.

I now realize that when I thought my life was at its bottom, my life was really perfect.

A single moment can change the course of your life. A single moment in time can destroy what you hold most dear. Some events in life leave you only two options: make the most of your life, doing something important to help others or the exact opposite, just let go and slip into that inky blackness of emotional abyss.

There is no middle ground to live a normal life. The death of my daughter was more than I could bear, but sometimes when your soul is sucked down a black hole, it is ejected out the other side.

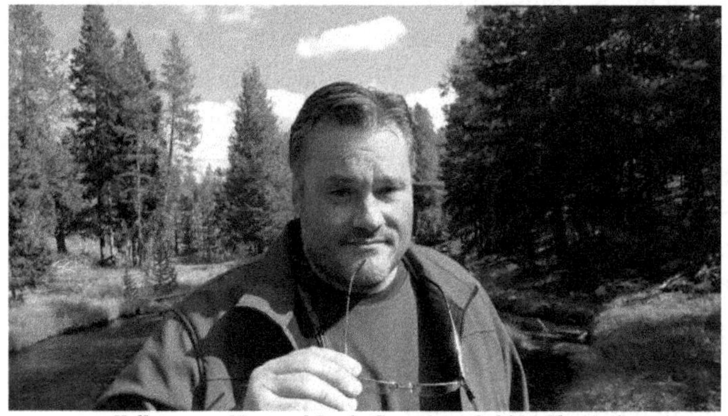

Yellowstone National Park. Copywrite © 2017 The Author

87

www.ingramcontent.com/pod-product-compliance
Lightning Source LLC
Chambersburg PA
CBHW070814280726
48660CB00015B/528